D0914742

MONOGRAPHS OF THE
INSTITUTE FOR THE STUDY OF
ANALGESIC AND SEDATIVE DRUGS

IV

ACETOPHENETIDIN

Monographs of the Institute for the Study of Analgesic and Sedative Drugs

I. ACETANILID: A Critical Bibliographic Review. By Martin Gross, M.D. New Haven; Hillhouse Press, 1946.

II. THE SALICYLATES: A Critical Bibliographic Review. By Martin Gross, M.D., and Leon A. Greenberg, Ph.D. New Haven; Hillhouse Press, 1948.

III. ANTIPYRINE: A Critical Bibliographic Review. By Leon A. Greenberg, Ph.D. New Haven; Hillhouse Press, 1950.

IV. ACETOPHENETIDIN: A Critical Bibliographic Review. By Paul K. Smith, Ph.D. New York; Interscience Publishers, Inc., 1958.

In Preparation

V. THE BROMIDES: A Critical Bibliographic Review. By Ebbe Curtis Hoff, Ph.D., M.D.

ACETOPHENETIDIN

A Critical Bibliographic Review

By **PAUL K. SMITH, Ph.D.**

Professor of Pharmacology
The George Washington University
School of Medicine

19 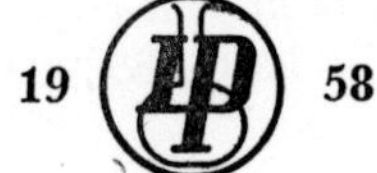 58

INTERSCIENCE PUBLISHERS

NEW YORK - LONDON

Published by arrangement with HILLHOUSE PRESS,
New Haven, Connecticut

Library of Congress Catalog Card Number 58-12721

INTERSCIENCE PUBLISHERS, INC., 250 Fifth Avenue, New York 1, N. Y.

For Great Britain and Northern Ireland:
INTERSCIENCE PUBLISHERS LTD., 88/90 Chancery Lane, London, W.C. 2

PRINTED IN THE UNITED STATES OF AMERICA BY
MACK PRINTING CO., EASTON, PENNSYLVANIA

Preface

The present monograph is the fourth in a series of critical reviews of the literature on analgesic and sedative drugs. The first volume dealt with acetanilid, the second with salicylates, the third with antipyrine; the fifth, now in preparation, deals with bromides.

The scientific press and research workers have received the earlier volumes generously, and it is to be hoped that the present one will be found to provide assistance in locating the scattered literature and in evaluating it. Perhaps the chief value of the work is to make available the pertinent literature in convenient form. Another, really no less important, is to aid future investigators by calling their attention to the inadequacies of past work so that these may be a guide to planning more definitive experiments in the future.

Recent work has shown that the major metabolite of acetophenetidin is *N*-acetyl-*p*-aminophenol. It appears likely that this substance also is responsible for the therapeutic activity of acetophenetidin. Since the pharmacology of these drugs is related so closely, it seemed advisable at this time to include in this volume reference to the increasing number of studies dealing with *N*-acetyl-*p*-aminophenol.

PAUL K. SMITH

Acknowledgments

The review of the literature and the preparation of this monograph were aided by a grant from the Institute for the Study of Analgesic and Sedative Drugs.

Drs. Raymond L. Conklin, Harvey B. Haag, Maurice H. Seevers, and McKeen Cattell very kindly read early drafts and offered a number of helpful suggestions. Dr. Claudia S. Prickett was most helpful in revising the manuscript.

The author is indebted to the staffs of the National Medical Library and the library of the The George Washington University School of Medicine for assistance in the search for references.

The author's colleagues, Drs. H. George Mandel, Gloria Comulada Feeney, Eberhard G. Trams, and Pierre Em. Carló, assisted with the translating.

A number of other associates helped with the abstracting and typing. Among them were: Theresa E. Capp, Ariel C. Hollinshead, Bette Kolonia, Julia M. Lampkin, Marilyn Ver Veer O'Toole, Eugenia Brandenburger Smith, and Katharine V. R. Smith.

I am indebted to Dr. Walter A. Compton for permission to refer to unpublished material from the Miles-Ames Laboratories.

Contents

Illustrations viii
Tables ix
Note on Reference Citations and on Use of the Bibliography . . . x
Abbreviations x
I. History 1
II. Physical and Chemical Properties 4
III. Estimation in Biological Material 7
IV. Fate of Acetophenetidin in the Body 8
V. Metabolism and Intermediary Products 15
VI. Antipyretic Action 20
VII. Analgesic Action 37
VIII. Other Therapeutic Uses 59
IX. Effects on Blood and Organ Systems 64
X. Toxicology 121
XI. Tolerance and Habituation 138
XII. Summary 141
Bibliography 149
Index 175

Illustrations

figure *page*

1. Plasma levels of acetophenetidin and metabolic products after the administration of 1.2 g. acetophenetidin to a normal man . . 9
2. Plasma levels of *N*-acetyl-*p*-aminophenol after oral administration with and without effervescent base to human subjects . . . 10
3. Metabolism of acetophenetidin showing its relation to *N*-acetyl-*p*-aminophenol 19
4. The antipyretic action of acetophenetidin and neocinchophen and their combination in rats 31
5. The increase in stimulant threshold for the tooth pulp of the rabbit after acetophenetidin 50
6. The average pain threshold elevation resulting from the administration of 0.3 g. acetophenetidin to normal human subjects . . 53
7. The analgesic effect of acetophenetidin, of a barbiturate, and of their combination in human subjects 55
8. Comparative analgesic effect in patients of *N*-acetyl-*p*-aminophenol and aspirin 57
9. The effect of daily administration of acetophenetidin, 250 mg. per kg., on the blood morphology of dogs 84
10. Species differences at maximum formation of methemoglobin for various doses of acetophenetidin 98
11. Mean values of methemoglobin in four subjects after the administration of 3 g. acetophenetidin or *N*-acetyl-*p*-aminophenol . . 100

Tables

table *page*

1. Solubility of acetophenetidin in several solvents 5
2. Distribution of acetophenetidin, *p*-phenetidin, and *N*-acetyl-*p*-aminophenol in dog tissues 12
3. The metabolic fate of acetophenetidin in man 18
4. Correlation of *p*-phenetidin and methemoglobin levels in the blood after administration of *p*-phenetidin and acetophenetidin to dogs. 97
5. Plasma acetophenetidin and per cent methemoglobin following oral administration of acetophenetidin to man 98
6. Acute toxic doses of acetophenetidin in various species of animals 135
7. Acute toxic doses of *N*-acetyl-*p*-aminophenol in various species of animals 136

Note on Reference Citations and on Use of the Bibliography

ORGANIZATION. The Bibliography is arranged alphabetically. Unsigned articles are listed in the Bibliography under Anonymous, except editorials which are listed under Editorial.

ABBREVATIONS. The names of periodicals have been abbreviated in accordance with the *List of Periodicals Abstracted by Chemical Abstracts* (American Chemical Society, The Ohio State University, Columbus 10, Ohio, 1956).

LANGUAGE OF REFERENCES. Titles in Danish, Dutch, English, French, German, Italian, Spanish, and Swedish are given in the original language. Titles from other languages have been translated into English.

Abbreviations

g.	gram(s)
gr.	grain(s)
kg.	kilogram(s)
mg.	milligram(s)
mg. per kg.	milligram(s) per kilogram of body weight
min.	minute(s)
ml.	milliliter(s)
mμ	millimicron(s)
μg.	microgram(s)
sec.	second(s)

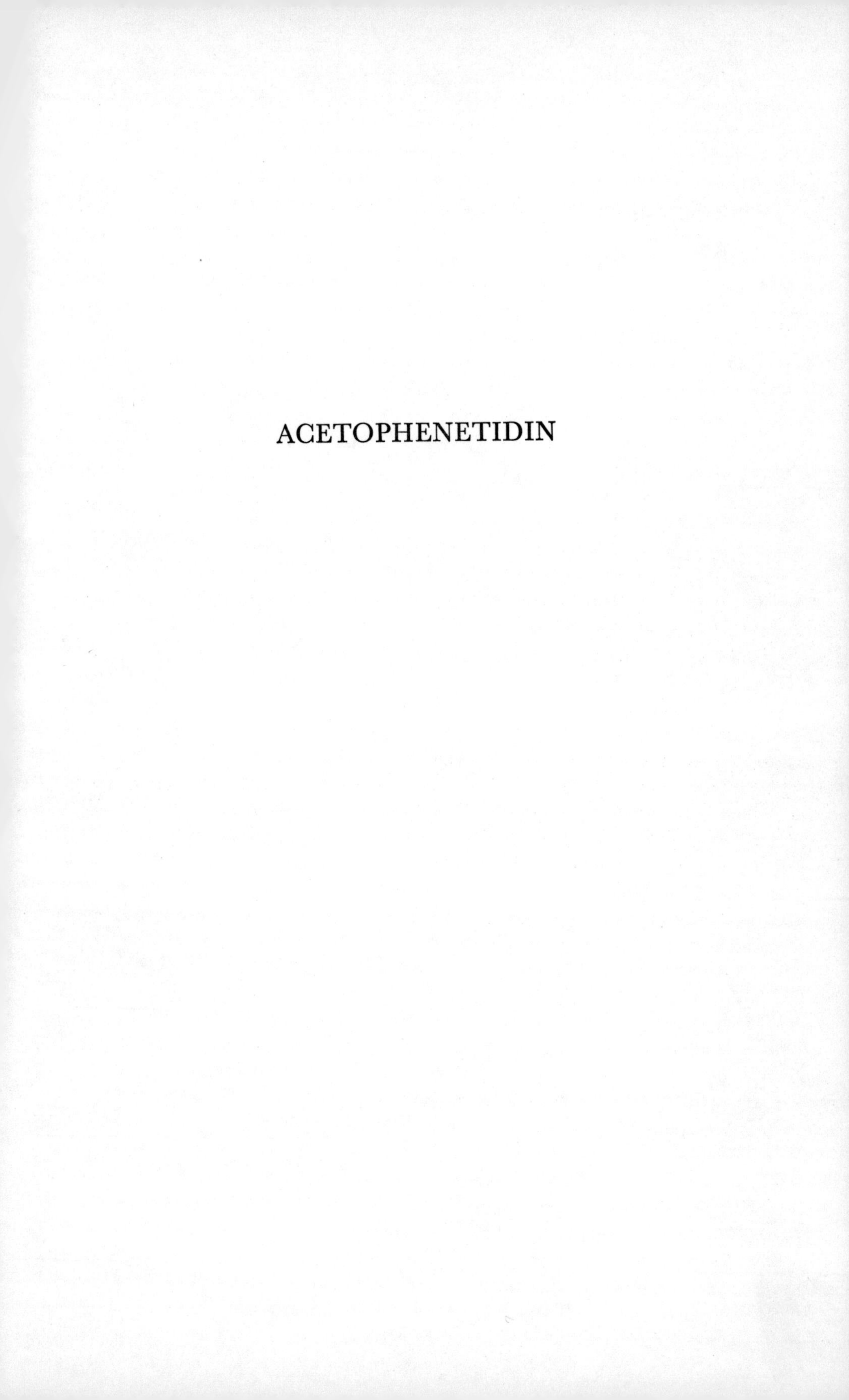

ACETOPHENETIDIN

Chapter I

History

Acetophenetidin was introduced into medical practice in 1887, only one after the accidental discovery of the therapeutic effects of acetanilid. The use of acetophenetidin as an antipyretic, however, was no accident, since it was appreciated from the beginning that it might prove to be effective for this purpose. Both drugs came at a time when it was believed that fevers invariably were harmful and should be relieved.

One of the earliest reports of the use of acetophenetidin is that of Hinsberg and Kast (206) in 1887. It is not clear that they were the first to employ it, since later (394) it is said that Kast and Bamberger were the first to use it as an antipyretic. Other reports of its use in 1887 pointed out its value in fevers and the relative absence of side-effects (206,245,246,271). One of its most vigorous proponents was Dujardin-Beaumetz (102,103). By 1888, one year after its introduction in Germany, there were reports of its use in England (24,27,165, 400), Scotland (27), Italy (68,371,419), France (102,103,117,144, 145,335,336,395,396), Russia (151), United States (211,359), Austria (228), Poland (261), and Bohemia (358). Knowledge of the use of acetophenetidin came rapidly to the United States; in 1888 we find Williams mentioning in the *American Journal of the Medical Sciences* (516) "the many reports on the use of phenacetin, or acetophenetidin. . . ."

It is of some interest that more than one-third of all the reports on acetophenetidin appeared before 1900. As was the case with so many drugs introduced in the last century or earlier, controlled pharmacological and clinical studies came later. Most frequently the effectiveness and absence of toxicity of acetophenetidin were assumed, and it was studied not so much to learn new facts about the drug itself as to provide a standard of comparison for the newer analgesic drugs. Perhaps an adequate impression of the early studies can best be obtained by considering some of the first reports.

Hinsberg and Kast did several studies of the toxicity of the drug in animals and tried it in patients. They observed that in fevers a temperature decrease of 2°C. could be obtained when the drug was administered in doses of 0.2 to 0.5 g. It was possible to suppress the rise in temperature which occurred in the evening or to postpone it. The fall in temperature proceeded slowly and reached a maximum at about 4 hours. After 3 or 4 hours the temperature rose again. Neither collapse nor cyanosis was observed following two to three 0.5-g. doses. The patients did not object to taking the drug because of its lack of taste and never experienced nausea, vomiting, or effect on the appetite during drug administration.

In the same year Lépine (271) described three main therapies for typhoid fever: the use of cold baths, the use of antipyretic drugs, and the use of intestinal antiseptics. He stressed the lack of toxicity of acetophenetidin, particularly the absence of cyanosis when used in doses of 0.5 g. six to eight times a day.

Köbler (245) described the use of acetophenetidin in the treatment of 50 patients with fever in a clinic in Vienna; of these, 11 had pulmonary tuberculosis, 10 had pneumonia, and 7 had typhus. He noted that acetophenetidin had no effect on the course of the diseases themselves. No intoxication other than marked decreases in body temperature was observed in these patients who received up to 1.6 g. per day, usually in doses of 0.7 g. Acetophenetidin had no undesirable effects on patients with nephritis. The usual fall in temperature with the doses employed was 1.5 to 2.5°C. It began about $^1/_2$ hour after administration of the drug and then continued at the rate of 0.1 to 0.2°C. per $^1/_4$ hour. When the maximum effect of a single dose had been obtained, the temperature rose gradually until after 8 to 10 hours the antipyretic effect had almost completely worn off. The decline in temperature after administration of the drug was steeper than its rise when the drug effect was wearing off. It produced the best results when given in the late afternoon and evening, and its action seemed to be additive with a physiological fever remission at that time of day. The antipyretic effect usually was not associated with perspiration, although there were patients who tended to sweat easily. No case of cyanosis or collapse was observed in any of these patients. Even in those cases of pneumonia in which the heart was affected the acetophenetidin was devoid of cardiac effects. The majority of patients who used acetophenetidin as an antipyretic became euphoric. Patients felt more at ease and the more spontaneous ones became talkative and exhibited an increase in appetite.

Köbler (246) observed that doses of 0.5 to 0.7 g. produced no decrease in temperature in normal subjects, whereas doses of 0.3 to 0.4 g. always produced a fall in temperature in patients with fever. If the drug was given at ten or twelve in the morning it usually would have to be given again in the afternoon. He concluded that the single administration of a large dose of from 0.5 and 0.7 g. was more effective than smaller individual hourly or 2-hourly doses. He never observed any side-effects such as nausea and vomiting, even though quantities of 0.6 to 0.7 g. were customarily employed. It had no detrimental effect on healing. He cites a total of 50 cases in which the drug was used.

An early champion of acetophenetidin as an analgesic antipyretic drug was Dujardin-Beaumetz (102,103). He pointed out that the cyanosis that occurred frequently after acetanilid and the skin eruptions and gastric upsets observed after antipyrine administration could be avoided by giving acetophenetidin. None of these toxic effects were observed with acetophenetidin, although in patients particularly sensitive to the drug with large doses of the order of 2 to 3 g. vertigo, drowsiness, and a feeling of cold were reported.

An early distributor of the drug, Schieffelin (417,418), summarized many of the first clinical observations and described some of the first animal experiments. A general description of its status in France in 1891 is given by Richelot *et al.* (394). Loebisch (286), in a book devoted to new drugs and their actions, reviews the early pharmacological and therapeutic work on acetophenetidin. Not all of the early reports were favorable. An anonymous writer in 1889 reports that the writers in England and in America were less impressed by the value of acetophenetidin, and that "Dr. Sidney Kinger has found it virtually useless in the wards of University College Hospital in London." As will be seen later there were at least two factors responsible for this: the failure to appreciate that acetophenetidin was not effective directly against the cause of fevers, and the tendency to use very large doses of the drug.

N-Acetyl-p-aminophenol. Perhaps the first investigator to use *N*-acetyl-*p*-aminophenol in therapy was von Mering (324) in 1893. Some of the early studies on it are reviewed by Von Oettingen (500). Its common use is of much more recent date. The demonstration that it is the major metabolite of acetophenetidin (45,48) as well as of acetanilid (47,161) and that it probably accounts for most or all of the therapeutic activity of acetophenetidin, stimulated clinical trials of the drug and led to its increased use.

Chapter II

Physical and Chemical Properties

Acetophenetidin is variously named *p*-ethoxyacetanilid and *N*-acetyl-*p*-phenetidine. Introduced as Phenacetin, this name has remained in common use. The structural formulas for it and for *N*-acetyl-*p*-aminophenol are:

$HN—CO—CH_3$ $HN—CO—CH_3$

OC_2H_5 OH

Acetophenetidin *N*-Acetyl-*p*-aminophenol

Acetophenetidin occurs as white, glistening crystals or as a fine, white crystalline powder with a melting point of 134–136°C. (493). One gram is soluble in 1300 ml. water, 15 ml. alcohol, 15 ml. chloroform, about 130 ml. ether, or 85 ml. boiling water. Its molecular weight is 179.2.

N-Acetyl-*p*-aminophenol, also known as *p*-hydroxyacetanilid, occurs as white crystals or as a fine, white crystalline powder with a melting point of 167–168°C. It is easily soluble in hot water, moderately soluble in ethanol, soluble in acetone, and relatively insoluble in cold water.

The original method of synthesis was essentially the same as that described by Schwyzer (428). The phenol was nitrated in the para position, the ethyl radical was introduced, and then the nitro group was reduced to the amino and acetylated. The details of the other methods of preparation from phenetidin are given by Manicke and Grigel (313). Wood *et al.* (523) described its preparation with the use of chlorobenzene as a starting material. Jenkins and Hartung (232) described its preparation from *p*-ethoxyphenol and benzene diazonium chloride with a subsequent reduction of the product to *p*-phenetidin. Swaminathan (475) discussed a new method of synthesizing acetophenetidin from phenol. The phenol was ethylated; then an acetyl group was introduced in a position para to the ethoxy group. The acetyl compound was converted to *p*-acetylphenetole oxime, which on treatment with phosphorous trichloride yielded acetophenetidin through a Beckman rearrangement.

Pinder and Venables (378) in 1938 found that, when acetophenetidin was prepared from *p*-phenetidin by acetylation with acetic acid, there was less tar formed if the reaction was carried out in an atmosphere of nitrogen instead of air. It was recognized very early that there were three possible isomers of acetophenetidin (111).

N-Acetyl-*p*-aminophenol was synthesized earlier than acetophenetidin. In 1878 Morse (343) mentioned that *N*-acetyl-*p*-aminophenol was produced during the reduction of *p*-nitrophenol with zinc and acetic acid, and that the acetic acid, instead of forming the acetate salt of the amine, produced acetylaminophenol. It crystallized in large white prisms of the monoclinic class with a melting point of 179°C.

Seidell (430) in 1907 published solubility measurements of acetophenetidin in a number of solvents. The results are given in Table 1.

TABLE 1
Solubility of Acetophenetidin in Several Solvents

Solvent	Temp., °C.	Solubility, g./100 g. solution
Water	25	0.11
Ether	25	1.56
Chloroform	25	4.76
Acetone	30–31	10.68
Benzene	30–31	0.65
Benzaldehyde	30–31	8.44
Amyl acetate	30–31	2.42
Aniline	30–31	9.46
Amyl alcohol	25	3.51
Acetic acid (99.5%)	21.5	13.65
Xylene	32.5	1.25
Toluene	25.0	0.30

Mandalá (311) in 1926 studied the solubility of acetophenetidin in water and in antipyrine solution at 14°C. The solubility in water was 0.054 per cent (0.000301 mole per liter); it was more than twice as great in a 10 per cent antipyrine solution.

In a study of the partition coefficients of a number of compounds between olive oil and water at 20°C., Macy (304) found that the partition coefficient of acetophenetidin was approximately 2.7 whereas that of acetanilid was 1.01.

Cramer (87) made vapor pressure measurements of acetophenetidin and expressed them as functions of temperature and pressure.

Kulkarni (259) has determined the dielectric constant and dipole moment of acetophenetidin at several temperatures. He has found that the dipole moment is abnormally high and suggests that it may be due to resonance effects.

Infrared measurements of acetophenetidin have been reported by Washburn and Kruger (507).

Occasionally acetophenetidin may have been adulterated intentionally. In a case described in 1890 (9) it was alleged that the druggist had added acetanilid to it, although the judge told the jury that adulteration for the sake of gain was out of the question. There is a notable incident (143) in which acetophenetidin was contaminated accidentally with *p*-chloroacetanilide with a resulting marked increase in toxicity.

Chapter III

Estimation in Biological Material

Adequate methods for determining acetophenetidin and its metabolic products in biological fluids were not devised until 1949, although most of the publications concerning the drug are prior to 1900. Early studies (307) described the excretion of the unchanged drug in the urine. These were based on a test for acetophenetidin in which, after digestion with hydrochloric acid and the addition of potassium dichromate and phenol, a brown color was obtained which turned blue on the addition of ammonia. The details of the use of this indophenol reaction for detecting acetophenetidin were given by Rohde (401).

In 1949 Goldbach and Opfer-Schaum (159) devised methods for the identification and isolation of acetophenetidin and other analgesics in tissues. The substances were extracted from the tissue with dilute sodium tungstate and the filtrate acidified and extracted with ether. After purification and the use of absorptive techniques and microsublimation, the substances were identified by micromethods including melting point and mixed melting point determinations.

An excellent method is the one devised by Brodie and Axelrod (48). In this method the biological material containing up to 10 mg. of acetophenetidin is extracted at pH 6 or higher with a mixture of isoamyl alcohol and benzene. The solvent phase is evaporated on a boiling water bath, and the residue, acidified with 0.5 *N* hydrochloric acid, is heated on a boiling water bath for 45 min. After cooling, the volume is adjusted with water, and the hydrolyzate diazotized with sodium nitrite solution. To develop color a solution of resublimed α-naphthol in alcohol is added, followed by sodium hydroxide. The dye is extracted with more of the isoamyl alcohol–benzene mixture to which is added a solution of trichloroacetic acid in ethylene dichloride. The optical density of the solution is measured at 600 mμ in a spectrophotometer adapted to microspectrophotometry. Standards are prepared by handling known amounts of the drug in the same manner as the unknown. Recovery of 1 to 5 μg. is 96 ± 5 per cent.

Chapter IV

Fate of Acetophenetidin in the Body

Absorption

Until recently the methods for the determination of acetophenetidin were not adequate to demonstrate how much drug was absorbed. Müller (345) reported that acetophenetidin was not changed by the acidic stomach contents or the alkaline pancreatic enzymes, but was absorbed unaltered. Lewin (276) stated that the compound was absorbed unchanged from the stomach. Neither author presented any evidence for this. Collischonn (81) used pastilles containing acetophenetidin and believed that there was sufficient absorption to produce analgesia. Evidence for its perlingual absorption based on its rapid analgetic action was given by Garbelli (146).

Only after the studies of Brodie and Axelrod (46,48) permitted differentiation of unchanged acetophenetidin from its metabolic products was it possible to show that a small amount of acetophenetidin was excreted in the urine of normal subjects. The stools were collected during the last 72 hours of administration and less than 1 per cent of the drug was recovered, indicating almost complete gastrointestinal absorption. The drug was not destroyed after incubation in stool suspensions for 24 hours at 30°C.

Albrecht (3) used suppositories consisting of aspirin, acetophenetidin, codeine phosphate, caffeine, and phenobarbital and believed that in infants the drug was absorbed more rapidly and was more effective by this route than when given orally in tablets.

It was observed by Carló *et al.* (63) that the addition of a mixture of citric acid and sodium bicarbonate resulted in a more rapid absorption of *N*-acetyl-*p*-aminophenol in human subjects when judged by plasma levels. Similarly, it was demonstrated by Davison *et al.* (93) that *N*-acetyl-*p*-aminophenol was rapidly absorbed from the stomach of the rat, and the rate was increased by the addition of sodium citrate.

Body Fluid Concentrations

Brodie and Axelrod (48) gave a dog 2.7 g. of acetophenetidin orally and 2 hours later killed the animal with an intravenous injection of air. They found that acetophenetidin, *p*-phenetidin, and *N*-acetyl-*p*-aminophenol were somewhat concentrated in the erythrocytes with smaller quantities in the cerebrospinal fluid. The plasma of the animal contained 57 mg. of acetophenetidin per liter while the red cells contained 60 mg. per kg., and the cerebrospinal fluid 36 mg. per liter.

When doses of 1.2 g. of acetophenetidin were given orally to a human subject, most of the drug was metabolized. At the end of 1 hour, there was approximately 0.7 mg. of the original drug per liter of plasma, and at the end of 2 hours there were 2.2 mg. This concentration gradually diminished until there was a negligible amount present at the end of 5 hours. Two other subjects were given 2 g. of drug. In one subject the peak plasma level was 4.9 mg. per liter at the end of 1 hour, and this slowly dropped to 0.2 mg. at the end of 8 hours. In the other, the maximum plasma level of 1.4 mg. per liter at the end of 1 hour decreased to 0.05 mg. per liter at the end of 5 hours. It is evident from this that there is considerable variation in the peak plasma levels obtained. Figure 1 presents some of these data.

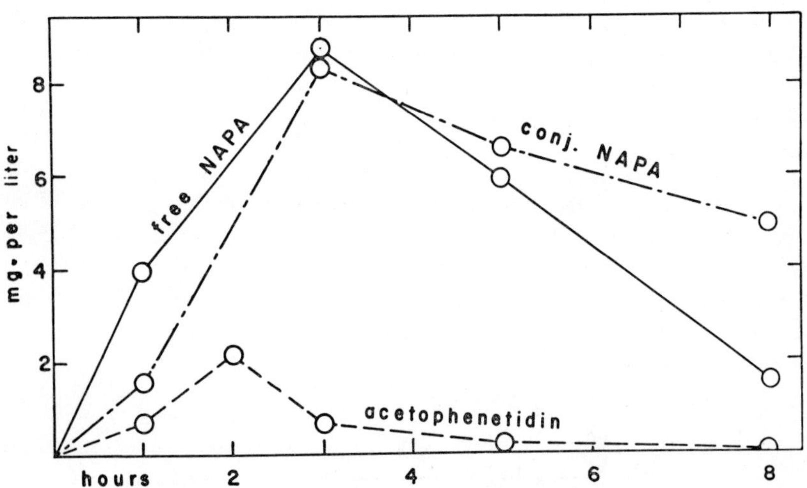

Figure 1. Plasma levels of acetophenetidin and metabolic products after the administration of 1.2 g. acetophenetidin to a normal man. (From Brodie and Axelrod, ref. 48.)

N-Acetyl-p-aminophenol

A dose of 0.5 g. *N*-acetyl-*p*-aminophenol in one human subject produced a serum level of 7.3 mg. per liter of the drug after 1 hour, and 4.2 mg. per liter in a second subject. The total conjugated drug in the serum was, respectively, 10.0 mg. per liter after 1 hour in the first case, and 10.2 mg. per liter after 2 hours in the second (74). One dog given 25 mg. per kg. had 8.1 mg. per liter in the serum 1 hour later, while another dog after 100 mg. per kg. had 76 mg. per liter.

When Brodie and Axelrod (44) gave human subjects 1 g. of *N*-acetyl-*p*-aminophenol, the peak plasma level after 2 hours was 8.2 mg. per liter in one case, and 10.9 mg. per liter in another. No detectable amount was present after 8 hours.

Carló *et al.* (63) administered *N*-acetyl-*p*-aminophenol to normal male subjects, giving the drug orally with a glass of water at least 6 hours after the last meal. Following doses of 0.3 g. *N*-acetyl-*p*-aminophenol, blood samples were drawn at 20, 40, 60, and 120 min. Later a dose of 0.6 g. was employed, and blood samples were taken at 15, 30, 90, and 150 min. Similar studies were made in which the drug was ingested along with an effervescent base. The results are illustrated in Figure 2. The blood plasma concentrations of *N*-acetyl-*p*-aminophenol obtained were approximately proportional to the

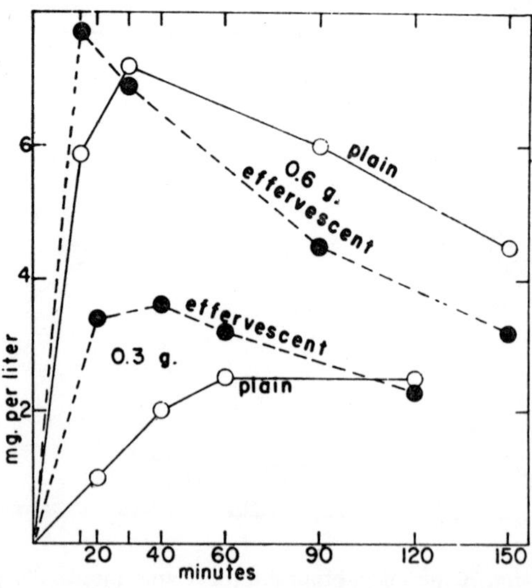

Figure 2. Plasma levels of *N*-acetyl-*p*-aminophenol after oral administration with and without effervescent base to human subjects. (From Carló *et al.*, ref. 63.)

dose given. It will also be noted that at 20 min. the average plasma values for the effervescent form were more than twice those for the ordinary form. They were still much higher for the former at 40 min. There was considerable variation in the individual responses, however, with three of the subjects showing quite low values at 20 min. after the effervescent form.

Distribution in Organs

It was not until the analytical methods for the determination of acetophenetidin were devised by Brodie and Axelrod (48) that it was possible to determine with accuracy the distribution of acetophenetidin in tissues. They gave 2.7 g. of acetophenetidin orally to a dog which they killed 2 hours later by an intravenous injection of air. The tissues were examined immediately, and the concentration of drug calculated in terms of tissue water. They found that acetophenetidin and its metabolic product, *p*-phenetidine, had concentrated in most of the tissues, while *N*-acetyl-*p*-aminophenol was fairly evenly distributed in terms of body water. The results are shown in Table 2. In addition, binding to plasma proteins was determined by dialysis against phosphate buffer at a pH of 7.4 at 37°C. with visking membranes as dialysis bags. Thirty per cent of the acetophenetidin and *p*-phenetidine and 25 per cent of the *N*-acetyl-*p*-aminophenol were bound to the plasma proteins at the levels of drug in the dog experiment. In a later study in the human and rat, it was demonstrated that at plasma levels of approximately 10 mg. per cent of *N*-acetyl-*p*-aminophenol more than half was bound to the plasma proteins (93).

Lester and Greenberg (275) studied the distribution of *N*-acetyl-*p*-aminophenol and its sulfuric acid ester between the erythrocytes and plasma when these were added to blood *in vitro*. In three separate experiments, the ratio of *N*-acetyl-*p*-aminophenol in cells to that in plasma was 1.3, 1.1, and 1.4, while there was no evidence that any of the sulfuric acid esters penetrated the erythrocytes. Presumably the distribution of the drug was not corrected for the difference in water content of blood and plasma.

Davison *et al.* (93) demonstrated in rats that the concentrations of *N*-acetyl-*p*-aminophenol in the brain were approximately the same as those found in the plasma at intervals of 30, 60, and 90 min. after oral administration.

TABLE 2

Distribution of Acetophenetidin, *p*-Phenetidin, and *N*-Acetyl-*p*-Aminophenol in Dog Tissues
(From Brodie and Axelrod, ref. 48)

Tissue	Acetophenetidin, mg./kg.	*p*-Phenetidin, mg./kg.	*N*-Acetyl-*p*-aminophenol, mg./kg.	Ratio: $\frac{\text{conc. in tissue water}}{\text{conc. in plasma water}}$		
				Acetophenetidin	*p*-Phenetidin	*N*-Acetyl-*p*-aminophenol
Plasma	57	12.3	96			
Red cells	60	13.5	96	1.60	1.70	1.50
C.S.F.	36	8.5	49	0.59	0.64	1.48
Liver	91	50.5	99	2.10	5.45	1.32
Kidney	67	26.5	104	1.40	2.62	1.29
Heart	56	19.2	79	1.21	1.89	1.00
Spleen	68	13.5	80	1.44	1.37	1.00
Lung	70	20.2	88	1.47	1.97	1.11
Brain	77	16.5	82	1.57	1.61	1.00
Muscle	48	17.1	69	1.05	1.74	0.90

Elimination

The first authors to publish studies concerning acetophenetidin, Hinsberg and Kast (206), reported that the drug and its degradation products were excreted in the urine of patients to whom the compound had been administered. Dujardin-Beaumetz (103) and Ott (359) noted that, within 1/2 hour after the administration of acetophenetidin, ferric chloride added to the urine gave a reddish-brown or black color. The studies of Ott were done on a normal healthy human male who was given 2 g. of the drug per day in three equal doses. Pesce (371) reported that after acetophenetidin administration the urine was intensely yellow and gradually assumed a reddish-brown color. Georgievsky (151) observed that after the administration of acetophenetidin the addition of ferric chloride to the urine produced first a reddish-brown color which later turned to a dark brown. He used this reaction to study the elimination of acetophenetidin in the urine. He found that it was present after 1/2 hour, reached its peak in 2 hours, lasted 3 to 4 hours, and then decreased in intensity. However, the ferric chloride test was still positive after 12 hours. Garcia y Mansilla (147) found that, in many, the drug was eliminated in the urine; its presence was demonstrated 20 min. after administration and as long as 24 hours later. Ubaldi (491,492) showed that in man there was an increase in the combined sulfuric acid in the urine after the ingestion of therapeutic amounts of acetophenetidin. The quantity used was a total of 3 g. in three doses at 4-hour intervals. That this increase was notable even after 24 hours was taken as proof of the slow excretion of the compound.

Storozhevoj (469) observed that the urine of a female patient about 16 years of age who had taken 25 g. of acetophenetidin in two doses on an empty stomach became a Burgundy wine color after the addition of ferric chloride. On standing it became black with a greenish tinge. The third day after the ingestion of the drug, the reaction with ferric chloride was weak, and on the fourth day it was negative, indicating that almost all of the drug had been excreted by that time. Hamill and Hine (176) found that a urine specimen collected the evening of the third day after a 37-year-old woman had taken an unknown number of acetophenetidin tablets gave no reaction for *p*-aminophenol. Even the specimen obtained 24 hours after the onset of symptoms gave no evidence of the breakdown products of acetophenetidin. On the other hand, the urine of a 1600-g.

albino rabbit, passed after it received an intraperitoneal injection of 0.35 g. of acetophenetidin, showed a well-marked reaction for *p*-aminophenol.

There has been very little work done upon the fecal excretion of unchanged acetophenetidin. Brodie and Axelrod (48) observed that when 2.0 g. of the drug was given daily in four divided doses for five consecutive days to normal human subjects less than 1 per cent of the dose was in the stools. They took this to indicate complete gastrointestinal absorption since the drug was not destroyed by incubating with the stools.

Although there are very few studies, the evidence is clear that acetophenetidin is readily absorbed from the gastrointestinal tract. Indirect evidence based on plasma levels also indicates that *N*-acetyl-*p*-aminophenol is absorbed well. Both acetophenetidin and *N*-acetyl-*p*-aminophenol enter into most of the cells of the body; there is a tendency for acetophenetidin to concentrate in some of the tissues but the concentration is usually no greater than twice that in the plasma water. *N*-Acetyl-*p*-aminophenol has a much more uniform distribution, showing no evidence of appreciable concentration in any tissue. The available data indicate that relatively lower concentrations of both drugs are found in the cerebrospinal fluid, but in the experiments reported there probably was inadequate time for equilibration. Data on their binding to the plasma proteins and on the relative concentrations in the brain and plasma lead, however, to the prediction that, even at equilibrium, their concentration in the cerebrospinal fluid would be appreciably less than in the plasma.

Chapter V

Metabolism and Intermediary Products

Shortly after acetophenetidin began to be used in therapy there appeared several studies of its metabolic fate. Most of the earlier studies were handicapped by a lack of precise analytical methods.

Hinsberg and Kast (206) observed that the urine of a patient who received 3 g. of the drug contained no free sulfate when tested with barium chloride. After boiling the sample with hydrochloric acid, however, they obtained an excellent precipitate with barium chloride, indicating a combined form of sulfate. If they refluxed the urine with concentrated hydrochloric acid for a time and then added phenol and potassium chromate, they obtained a brown-red color which turned a green-blue upon the addition of ammonia. Acetophenetidin gave the test only after boiling with hydrochloric acid. Since phenetidin gave the color without boiling it was concluded that, in addition to the unchanged acetophenetidin, phenetidin also was present in the urine. They further observed that when a dog had received 3 g. of acetophenetidin orally, there appeared in the urine a substance which readily reduced alkaline copper solution.

It was not until much later (441) that this reaction was shown to be due to the presence of a glucuronide, which is a major metabolite of acetophenetidin in the rabbit, and presumably in the dog as well.

Müller (345–347) observed that the drug was not excreted unchanged by the human but appeared in the urine as phenetidin, whose presence could be demonstrated in an alkaline ether extract of urine by means of diazo formation. This was accomplished by first treating the urine with 2 or 3 drops of hydrochloric acid, and then adding alkaline α-naphthol solution until the mixture was basic, at which point a red color appeared. Subsequent addition of hydrochloric acid produced a violet color. Ferric chloride added to the urine of patients who had received acetophenetidin produced a red-violet color, probably due to phenetidin which became dark green when the sample was shaken. Chromic acid and other oxidizing agents produced colors similar to the ones obtained with ferric chloride. Müller further observed that with increasing doses increasing amounts of conjugated sulfate appeared in the urine. After acetophenetidin administration the urine was *levo*-rotatory and this effect too increased with the dose (346).

Since the urine reduced alkaline copper oxide solution, but gave a negative fermentation test, he assumed that it also contained a conjugate of glucuronic acid. He concluded that aniline probably was not formed from acetophenetidin in the body and for that reason the drug was safer to use than other available antipyretics. He did believe, however, that a patient with a fever produced an additional metabolite or metabolites; a crystalline red dye, which gave a violet color with concentrated sulfuric acid, could be isolated from the urine of febrile patients treated with the drug. He also noticed an increase in the conjugated sulfate excretion after acetophenetidin.

Mörner (341,342) gave patients acetophenetidin and isolated the ethereal sulfate of *N*-acetyl-*p*-aminophenol from the urine. Hare (182) gave a dog as much as 3 g. of acetophenetidin and observed that the urine gave a Fehling's sugar reaction. Ubaldi (491,492) gave three 1-g. doses of acetophenetidin, one every 4 hours, to human subjects and observed a marked rise in urinary sulfate. The increase was notable even 24 hours later, which he took as proof of the slow excretion of the compound. After high doses of acetophenetidin he could not, however, demonstrate an increase in glucuronide by an increase in reducing substance as Müller had done. He also observed increased sulfate excretion in a dog after giving the animal 1 g. of the drug. Lewin (276) believed that acetophenetidin was secreted in the urine as phenetidin but he presented no evidence for this view. One of the early investigators of acetophenetidin (486) concluded that since the urine of patients receiving the drug gave the indophenol reaction, acetophenetidin had been converted either to *p*-aminophenol or to *N*-acetyl-*p*-aminophenol. Baccarani (20) gave 3 g. a day to patients and observed that there was a notable increase in the elimination of sulfuric ethers which lasted for some time after drug intake ceased. Edlefsen (113) was unable to confirm the results of Müller regarding the presence of phenetidin in the urine after the administration of phenacetin. It appears that Müller used a patient who had received much acetophenetidin for a long period of time whereas Edlefsen had given smaller doses for a shorter period of time.

As late as 1955, Wuhrmann and Jasinski (525) attributed the formation of methemoglobin following the chronic administration of acetophenetidin to *p*-aminophenol and hydroxylamine, but they presented no evidence that these were actual intermediary products. As will be seen, there is considerable reason to believe that they are not.

Bernheim (30) discussed the hydrolysis of acetophenetidin suspensions. The enzyme responsible for the hydrolysis was an acylase, one of a group of enzymes known to hydrolyze acetylated amino acids, and its specificity was tested with various compounds. When the rate of hydrolysis of acetanilid was assigned a value of 100, the value for acetophenetidin was 14. He thought that the rate of hydrolysis found for acetophenetidin was probably less than the true rate because of the slight solubility of the drug.

Smith and Williams (440) speculated that the activity of acetophenetidin could be explained by its slow conversion *in vivo* into *N*-acetyl-*p*-aminophenol. Brodie and Axelrod (45) studied the route of metabolism of acetophenetidin and found that a major fraction was de-ethylated to form *N*-acetyl-*p*-aminophenol. They gave subjects 1 to 2 g. and showed that about 0.2 per cent of this was excreted as the unchanged drug, 0.1 per cent as *p*-phenetidin, 3.5 per cent as *N*-acetyl-*p*-aminophenol, and about 74 per cent as conjugated *N*-acetyl-*p*-aminophenol. Using the precise analytical methods that they developed, Brodie and Axelrod (48) then made more complete studies of the fate of the drug. As may be seen from Table 3, very little unchanged drug is excreted, and most of it is converted to conjugated *N*-acetyl-*p*-aminophenol. More recently Brodie *et al.* (49) have shown that acetophenetidin is de-ethylated rapidly to *N*-acetyl-*p*-aminophenol by an enzyme system from rabbit liver microsomes. The reaction was enhanced by nicotinamide, triphosphopyridine nucleotide, magnesium ions, and glucose-6-phosphate. There was little activity in the nuclei or mitochondria. The reaction was inhibited by diethylamino-ethyldiphenylpropylacetate. The species differences in the cleavage of acetophenetidin at the ethoxy group has been described by Axelrod (17).

Smith and Williams (441) gave acetophenetidin orally in doses of 0.3 to 0.7 g. per kg. to rabbits and studied its metabolic products. The major metabolic change was de-ethylation, followed by conjugation, mostly with glucuronide, but to some extent with sulfate. By isolation of the *p*-acetamidophenylglucuronide, they demonstrated

TABLE 3
The Metabolic Fate of Acetophenetidin in Man (48)

Drug administered, g.	Acetophenetidin, %	*p*-Phenetidin, %	*N*-Acetyl-*p*-aminophenol, %	Conjugated *N*-Acetyl-*p*-aminophenol, %
1.0	0.17	0.12	3.5	82
1.2	0.36	0.02	4.7	65
2.0	0.15	0.04	3.1	80
2.0	0.30	0.15	3.6	81
2.0	0.23	0.03	2.6	81
2.0	0.23	0.13	3.9	57

that approximately 47 per cent of the drug was excreted in this form. They estimated that an additional 7 per cent of the drug was excreted as the ethereal sulfate. They concluded that deacetylation took place only to a slight extent since very little free *p*-phenetidin, on the order of 0.1 per cent of the administered dose, could be detected in the urine.

N-Acetyl-p-aminophenol. In a later study, Smith and Williams (442) showed that *N*-acetyl-*p*-aminophenol, when given in a dose comparable to that of acetophenetidin on a molecular basis, was excreted by rabbits 63 per cent as glucuronide and 10 per cent as ethereal sulfate. There was no compound in the urine containing diazotizable amino groups. Later they (443) demonstrated that *N*-acetyl-*p*-aminophenol could be formed from phenetidin, which was acetylated to acetophenetidin and then de-ethylated to *N*-acetyl-*p*-aminophenol. The mechanism they believed likely was the conversion of phenetidin to acetophenetidin, and then to *N*-acetyl-*p*-aminophenol, and finally to its glucuronide.

In an attempt to determine whether *N*-acetyl-*p*-aminophenol is deacetylated and later reacetylated *in vivo*, Smith *et al.* (450) gave several species of animals acetyl-labeled drug and studied the relative radioactivity of the urinary metabolites. In monkeys and in one human subject there was evidence of appreciable exchange of acetyl groups, but in rabbits, cats, and one human subject there was no significant exchange.

The development of precise analytical methods has made it possible to determine that the major portion of acetophenetidin is de-ethylated to *N*-acetyl-*p*-aminophenol. Very little of it is converted

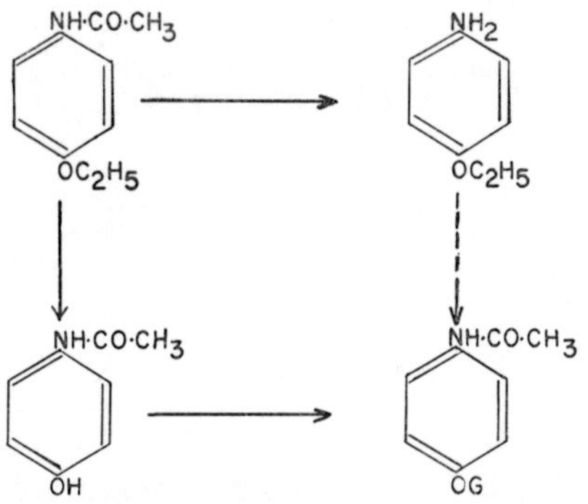

$NH \cdot CO \cdot CH_3$ → NH_2

OC_2H_5 OC_2H_5

$NH \cdot CO \cdot CH_3$ → $NH \cdot CO \cdot CH_3$

OH OG

Figure 3. Metabolism of acetophenetidin showing its relation to *N*-acetyl-*p*-aminophenol. (The symbol G represents glucuronic acid or sulfuric acid.)

to *p*-phenetidin. Only small amounts of the drug are excreted unchanged, most of it being excreted as a conjugated form of *N*-acetyl-*p*-aminophenol. Figure 3 is a diagram illustrating the metabolism of acetophenetidin and its relation to *N*-acetyl-*p*-aminophenol.

Chapter VI

Antipyretic Action

Clinical Observations

Few drugs have been as readily accepted into general use as acetophenetidin. Coming in an era when fevers were usually treated with drugs, it was quickly recognized that acetophenetidin was worthy of a place among the accepted remedies of that day.

Since the first therapeutic use of acetophenetidin was as an antipyretic, it is not surprising that most of the early reports concerned this action of the drug. It was reported by Richelot *et al.* (394) that in 1887 Kast and Bamberger (237) were the first to use it as an antipyretic. Hinsberg and Kast (206) observed that it was a good antipyretic in tuberculous patients, causing the temperature to fall about 2°C. when administered in doses of 0.2 to 0.5 g. The temperature decreased slowly and reached a minimum at about 4 hours. There were no violent symptoms or unusual secretion of sweat, and the skin was only slightly red. Köbler (245) observed that doses of 0.3 to 0.4 g. always produced a fall in temperature in febrile patients whereas the same dose had no effect on normal subjects. Even doses of 0.5 to 0.7 g. did not reduce the body temperature of normal subjects, although in patients with a temperature of 39.5 to 40.5°C. the same quantity of drug usually produced a fall of 1.5 to 2.5°C. This drop in temperature, beginning 1/2 hour after administration of the drug, then continued at about 0.1 to 0.2°C. per 1/4 hour. When the maximal effect had been reached, the temperature rose gradually until 8 to 10 hours later the drug effect had completely worn off. Köbler's work attracted attention early in England (6). In the United States, Mays (320) obtained a small amount of the drug and used it in tuberculous patients in whom he found it to be an effective antipyretic.

When acetophenetidin first became available, it was tried in many different types of fever associated with a number of different diseases. Lépine (271) described its use in the treatment of typhoid fever. He used 0.5 g. six to eight times a day.

An early British report is that of Carslaw (64) who, in most cases, administered 0.3 to 0.6 g. doses of acetophenetidin. Usually he obtained a prompt decrease in the temperature of patients suffering from tuberculosis. Cattani (68) noted that in the normal individuals perspiration was not observed after the administration of acetophenetidin but in febrile cases perspiration sometimes was very abundant. The lowering of body temperature did not correspond in time with the occurrence of maximum perspiration. In 61 cases representing a variety of diseases, the usual dose he employed was 0.4 to 0.7 g. Dujardin-Beaumetz (103) observed that the average dose of 0.3 g. produced a fall in temperature of 3°C. in tuberculosis and typhoid fever. The action of the drug started in about 20 min. and lasted from 8 to 10 hours. Gaiffe (144,145) observed that in the therapeutic use of the drug the antipyretic action was maximal in about 4 hours and disappeared after 8 to 10 hours. Georgievsky (151) observed that patients given 0.2 to 0.3 g. usually had a fall in temperature of about 0.5°C. in the first 1/2 hour. Their temperature continued to decrease gradually, but in 2 to 3 hours it had reached a minimum. Then climbing gradually, the temperature returned to its previous height 8 to 10 hours after intake of the drug. Grenfell (165) observed that acetophenetidin, in doses of 0.5 g. given to the average adult, was successful as an antipyretic in pleurisy, pneumonia, and tuberculosis. Guttmann (168) used acetophenetidin for several months and stated that it was a very strong antipyretic, stronger even than antipyrine, and effective in doses of 0.5 g. Heusner (205) noted that after administration of 1 g. of acetophenetidin there was a fall in body temperature which lasted from 8 to 10 hours and was accompanied by slight sweating. If the latter effect was inhibited by atropine, the temperature drop was less. He observed that 1 g. of acetophenetidin was equivalent to 0.5 g. of acetanilid or 2.0 g. of antipyrine as an antipyretic. Hirshfelder (209) reported that as an antipyretic the drug produced sweating 30 to 50 minutes after administration, the usual antipyretic effect beginning 1 to 2 hours after administration and reaching its peak in the 4th hour. The temperature rose to a maximum after another 6 hours. The drug had no effect on normal temperature but did produce mild sweating.

Hoppe (215) first gave himself 0.2 g. of the drug without any effect. When he took 0.4 g. he had slight sweating underneath the arms and around the navel while sitting still at a table, but with doses of 0.6 to 1.0 g. he did not observe any perspiration. His temperature dropped only very little after 1.0 g., and he felt slight chills which lasted about 1/2 hour. Doses of 1.5 g. produced a lack of concentrating ability as if he had drunk several glasses of beer. They also produced yawning. He felt pressure in the forehead, and his eyelids burned and became heavy. His temperature fell from 36.8 to 36.55°C., and the pulse rate went down slightly. An hour after taking the drug these symptoms had ceased. Another hour later he felt well with a normal temperature. When he took 2 g. on two successive days he had even fewer symptoms.

Hoppe then gave a dose of 1.25 g. to a girl slightly anemic in appearance to find out what the effects would be on the central nervous system. After a quarter of an hour he observed slight shaking, chills, eructation, yawning, sleepiness, and difficulty in concentrating. These symptoms lasted only 1/2 hour, but the tiredness remained. The temperature of the patient dropped 0.3°C. Later when 1 g. was given for headaches there were no side-effects. In a 40-year-old woman with migraine, 1 g. of acetophenetidin produced symptoms similar to those shown in the preceding except for the chills and dizziness, but the migraine was improved. If Hoppe repeated the dose the same symptoms recurred. When the first dose did not remove her headache, he gave a second one 4 hours later. Twenty minutes after this he observed dizziness and tiredness, followed in 5 min. by shaking in the limbs. Still a few minutes later there was a stomach disturbance and very heavy yawning; then the nails of her fingers became blue, and there was some nausea. Within 10 min. of this there was some improvement, and 35 min. later the patient felt well.

Hoppe concluded that acetophenetidin was relatively nontoxic, and although it might produce individual reactions, these were not severe. These reactions appeared mostly in weak and anemic people and usually were over 2 to 3 hours after the drug was given. He also observed that in children doses of 0.125 g. produced a fall in temperature of 1.5 to 2.0°C. Doses of 0.2 to 0.25 g. usually were sufficient to drop the temperature to normal in the late afternoon. Doses of 0.4 g. were well tolerated by a 7-year-old girl with a high fever whose temperature fell from 40.5 to 36.8°C. in 4 hours. He observed that the main action of the drug occurred from 2 to 4 hours after its administration. After that the temperature rose slowly. The total duration of action was from 2 to 8 hours.

Lachowicz (261), observing a number of cases of various types of fevers, found that acetophenetidin was an effective antipyretic, with a dose of 0.5 g. producing a fall in temperature of 1.5 to 3°C. Mahnert (307,308) found that he could give doses of 0.9 g. two to three times a day without untoward effects. Doses of 0.9 g. of acetophenetidin as an antipyretic were equivalent to 1 g. of quinine or 2 g. of sodium salicylate. He believed that acetanilid acted more rapidly and more intensively than acetophenetidin but that its action was not as prolonged. Masius (319) studied the effects of acetophenetidin in 7 cases of typhoid fever and found that the antipyretic effect was irregular. He observed no striking results in 5 cases of pulmonary tuberculosis and only a rather weak effect in 4 cases of pneumonia.

Müller (345–347) found that in patients with typhus, erysipelas, puerperal fever, and tuberculosis doses of 0.5 to 0.75 g. of acetophenetidin lowered temperatures to normal at once. Seldom were doses of 1.0 g. necessary. A maximal decrease in temperature was reached in 1 to 4 hours. The apyrexia lasted for 2 to 5 hours, and then the temperature rose again. Concomitant with the fall in temperature there was sweating, but this was not a serious side-effect. Usually there were no chills during these events. In some cases the patients received as much as 6 to 8 g. of drug per day, with no evidence of collapse or side-effects.

Péréra (369) used acetophenetidin in cases of pneumonia. He gave two doses of 0.25 g. and in 10 hours the temperature fell from 40 to 37°C. Also, in a case of bronchitis in a 2-month-old infant he obtained complete calm after giving 0.15 g. divided into two doses. Pesce (370) observed that acetophenetidin was a good antipyretic and improved the general condition of the patient. The usual decrease in the temperature of febrile patients given 0.5-g. he obtained complete calm after giving 0.15 g. divided into two doses was 2 to 3°C. Doses of 0.5 g. (371), according to him, corresponded in their antipyretic effect to 1.0 g. of antipyrine or 0.25 g. of acetanilid. It was sometimes necessary to give individual doses of 0.5 to 0.7 g. at one time, but he thought this was better than successive smaller doses at short intervals. The lowering of the temperature started 30 to 45 min. after the drug was administered and reached its climax in 3 to 5 hours. Even after 8 hours there was an appreciable decrease in body temperature which then rose slowly again to its original value. Rohden (402) usually gave doses of

0.15 to 1.0 g. to adults and 0.05 to 0.2 g. to children, but in some cases he employed just 1 g. in a single dose. The antipyretic effect began in $^1/_2$ hour. Rifat (396) gave doses of 0.3 g. and observed that the temperature fell after 1 to $1^1/_2$ hours. The effect did not last beyond 3 hours, so he had to give a second dose after 4 hours. Rifat (395) found acetophenetidin to be effective for relief of pain but inferior to antipyrine as an antipyretic.

Rumpf (406) usually gave adults 1 g. as a single dose but observed that frequently 0.5 g. was sufficient. For children he used 0.2 to 0.25 g. Suckling (473) found the drug to be equal to antipyrine in its actions against fever, and without disagreeable after effects. Warfvinge (504) reported the successful use of acetophenetidin in doses of 0.5 to 1.0 g. as an antipyretic in 59 patients, most of them with typhoid fever. Zannas (528) found the drug to be an effective antipyretic.

Ayers (18) showed that 0.7 g. of acetophenetidin was sufficient to lower high temperatures 3°C. within 2 to 4 hours. The fall usually began not more than 30 min. after drug administration.

Burkhalter (58) found that 0.5 g. was adequate for optimal antipyresis and that a single dose of 0.5 g. was more effective than multiple small doses of 0.12 or 0.2 g. The drug was administered no more than once or twice a day. The antipyretic effect began about $^1/_2$ hour after administration with the greatest decrease in temperature occurring in 2 to 5 hours. Sometimes the temperature dropped below the normal value from 6 to 9 hours after the drug had been given. He concluded that acetophenetidin produced a longer antipyretic effect than a cold bath. Crombie (89) compared the antipyretic effect of antipyrine, acetanilid, and acetophenetidin in cases of dysentery and acute pneumonia. He concluded that acetophenetidin had the advantage that, in cases where the fever was complicated with unrest and insomnia, even doses of 0.1 to 0.3 g. produced sleep without headache the following morning. Dujardin-Beaumetz (105) observed that the lowering of body temperature was most notable in cases of fever, doses of 0.5 g. causing a fall of 1.0 to 2.0°C. This action lasted 4 hours and was accompanied by profuse sweating.

Gates (149) selected two patients suffering from a fever due to chronic tuberculosis and gave them several different drugs successively for a varying number of days. One of the patients had an average daily temperature fluctuation of 1.8°C. without treatment.

The exact order with which he gave the drugs was not recorded. For the daily dose of 1.3 g. acetanilid, the average daily temperature variation was 0.44°C., with acetophenetidin in doses of 0.4 to 0.8 g. it was 0.64°C., and with antipyrine, 0.82°C. When he gave acetophenetidin again he observed a fluctuation of 1.08°C. At other times with doses of 0.7 to 0.8 g. of acetophenetidin this was 1.17°C., and with 0.5 g. it was 1.96°C. This author concluded that the most effective antipyretic drug was acetanilid in dosage of 1.2 g. a day in four equal doses, and that acetophenetidin, 0.8 g. a day in divided doses, was next, while antipyrine in a dose of 1.0 g. a day was third.

Geisler (150) gave 0.5 g. doses to patients with fever and observed decreases in temperature as great as 2°C. In 1889 Horváth (219, 220) was one of the first to report the use of acetophenetidin in Hungary. He gave not more than 3 g. a day for fever and usually obtained a decrease in temperature of 0.3 to 0.56°C. after doses of 0.125 to 0.5 g. After 3 to 4 hours the average fall in temperature was 1.5 to 2.5°C. The temperature was normal again after 6 to 8 hours. He also described observations on 25 middle-aged adult patients whose temperatures had either reached or surpassed 39°C. In the beginning he gave doses of 0.125 to 0.25 g. but later increased them to 1 g. Usually small doses produced a fall in body temperature of 0.3 to 0.5°C. within 1 hour accompanied by moderate sweating, and at the end of 3 to 4 hours the temperature had fallen 1.5 to 2.5°C. Following this there was a slow rise until in 6 to 8 hours the temperature was back to its original level. In a few cases as little as 0.125 g. was sufficient to obtain considerable and occasionally complete remission of the fever.

There were early discussions on the use of the drug as an antipyretic, such as those of Huet (223), in which no data were given. Humphreys (224), in a limited experience, found that 0.15 g. coated pills of acetophenetidin were excellent as an antipyretic. In 1889 Pesce and Assauto (372) reported a series of cases in which they had followed the temperature curves in various diseases after the administration of doses of acetophenetidin of the order of 1 g. Specker (461) concluded that in normal subjects acetophenetidin had no effect on the body temperature but was a powerful antipyretic in the presence of fever, its effects beginning at 1 hour, reaching a maximum after 2 hours, and lasting a total of 5 or 6 hours. Tripold (488) observed that with doses of 0.2 g. in children there were no disagreeable effects but only a pronounced antipyretic one.

Ayers (19) considered acetophenetidin an antipyretic *par excellence,* better than antipyrine or acetanilid. He found that 0.5 g. lowered the temperature 1.7°C., and in continued fevers he repeated the dose every 4 to 6 hours. Garcia y Mansilla (147) showed that the antipyresis after administration of acetophenetidin began in 1/2 hour and continued with oscillations for 4 hours, by which time the maximal effect was observed. The temperature then began to rise until it approached its original level 8 hours after the drug was administered. Espinosa (121) conducted clinical trials substituting acetophenetidin for antipyrine which he found had caused collapse in typhus patients. It will be remembered that collapse of typhus patients may occur when they are not receiving drugs. Initially he gave 0.3 g. doses but noticed no lowering in the temperature within 1 hour. After 2 or 3 days he raised the dose to 0.5 g. in the morning and afternoon and observed that, even so, the temperature always fell slowly. Kartschewski (236), in several cases of abdominal typhus, found that acetophenetidin produced a marked decrease in temperature followed by a rise, sometimes accompanied by chills. Sommer (458) mentions that acetophenetidin in a typhus epidemic in Russia proved to be effective in reducing the fever and produced general improvement without disagreeable side-effects. He gave the drug, 0.2 g. for children and 0.4 g. for adults, three or four times a day.

Demme (94) said that acetophenetidin was a good antipyretic but without any specific effect on the cause or processes of the disease. Large doses of the drug produced a prompt effect compared to multiple small doses. Hare (182) believed that it lowered the body temperature by decreasing heat production, and that there was even a slight decrease in the rate of heat loss. MacGillycuddy (295), in a short note, mentioned that he had used the drug successfully as an antipyretic for the past two years.

Caldwell (62) discussed the manner of fever reduction, and although he realized that knowledge of mechanism at that time was very rudimentary, he expressed the opinion that acetophenetidin, salicylic acid, antipyrine, and acetanilid reduced temperature mainly by depressing the thermoregulatory center. Cleaves (75) preferred to use cold sponging and cold baths to combat fever. He considered that all drugs, such as salicylates, antipyrine, acetanilid, and acetophenetidin produced their antipyretic effect by direct action on the constituents of the blood, to limit the oxidative processes, and by depression of the nerve centers, either to decrease production of or to increase dissipation of heat. Ott (360) discussed the antipyretics in use at that time, including acetophenetidin, but he gave no original data. Several compounds, derivatives of *p*-aminophenol closely related to acetophenetidin, are discussed by von Mering (324). He believed that *N*-acetyl-*p*-aminophenol produced the same side-reactions as *p*-aminophenol. In his opinion acetophenetidin was one of the least toxic of the compounds, and he mentioned its use in 5 patients with fever.

In a textbook on new drugs, Loebisch (286) discussed acetophenetidin and gave quite a number of the earlier references to its analgesic and antipyretic activities. Thomson (479) believed that acetophenetidin was not as satisfactory as a combination of acetanilid and antipyrine, 0.3 g. of each, administered as a dry powder with a mouthful of water. Acetophenetidin seemed to quiet nervous patients without controlling fever.

Eldridge (116) used acetophenetidin in typhoid fever, malaria, influenza, pneumonia, gonorrheal rheumatism, and tuberculosis. The doses employed were relatively large. The fevers abated and speedy recoveries ensued with no complications.

Biernacki (34) used 0.15-g. doses of acetophenetidin every 4 hours in 20 cases of enteric fever without noticeable result beyond varying oscillations in the temperature. While the temperature was down the skin was usually pale and clammy. As a rule, the temperature rose again within 4 hours after the drug was given, and even exceeded its original level.

Shlenker (434) found the antipyretic effects of acetophenetidin and methoxyaceto-*p*-phenetidin in pulmonary tuberculosis to be comparable.

Brunton (56), in summarizing the status of acetophenetidin, said that it was a powerful antipyretic, producing rapid sweating, with an action very much like that of antipyrine, but less depressing. He believed that sometimes it lowered the temperature so quickly that it took away the stimulus to the heart which was provided by the circulating blood. Cmuchal (77) gave patients doses of 0.5 to 1.0 g. and observed that, regardless of the cause of the fever, the drug was an effective antipyretic. Frazer (137) classified antipyretics as those which control the circulation and those which control the secretions and excretions, especially of the sweat glands. He placed quinine, antipyrine, acetanilid, and acetophenetidin in this latter category.

While Warner (505) recommended acetophenetidin as an antipyretic in influenza, he thought it should be used only for a limited period, since long use might weaken the heart. Long (289) advocated combating fever by hydrotherapy, but did use antipyretics during 9 to 10 years of practice without ill effects, and considered acetophenetidin less depressing than acetanilid. In cases of pneumonia with high temperature, accompanied by restlessness and rapid breathing, prompt relief was afforded by one or two doses of acetophenetidin. When used in inflammatory rheumatism it was combined with salicylate.

Löbl (285) observed a law student who became quite ill after taking two powders containing 0.5 g. of acetophenetidin. He had an axillary temperature of 35.2°C. He perspired freely, and 6 hours later his temperature had risen to 36.3°C. though the chills had ceased. In another case, Storozhevoj (469) reported a girl 18 years of age who had taken 25 g. of acetophenetidin in two doses on an empty stomach. She became ill immediately and, when observed, her body temperature under the axilla was 35.3°C. In a number of cases of typhus acetophenetidin reduced the temperature to about the same extent as the other antipyretics, but its duration of action was longer, antipyresis lasting about 4 to 6 hours and occasionally even 8 to 10 hours. The usual dose in adults was 0.5 g.

Acetophenetidin-Containing Mixtures. At the time acetophenetidin came into use, several other antipyretic agents were already being employed. Some early reports tell of the use of acetophenetidin combined with one or more of these.

Pierce (377) used a mixture of acetophenetidin and phenyl salicylate, 0.15 g. of each, and found that the antipyretic effects began in 30 to 45 min. and were maximal in 4 hours. He stated "phenacetine . . . has already gained such a foothold with the profession, that a permanent place in the future materia-medica might quite safely be predicted for it." He said further "its praises are sung by every medical journal throughout the land."

Haller (174) found that a mixture of phenyl salicylate and acetophenetidin, 0.15 g. of each, every 3 hours, shortened the duration of pain and fever in 314 cases of influenza.

Eldridge (115) prescribed 0.2 g. acetophenetidin plus 0.15 g. of quinine sulfate in capsules every 3 hours for influenza. This mixture given in the afternoon usually controlled typhoid fever, especially the severe headache, and permitted a restful night.

Busch (60) discussed the merits of a mixture of 0.05 g. caffeine, with 0.015 g. each of acetophenetidin, phenyldimethylpyrazine, and dimethylaminophenazone. He used it in approximately 100 cases of gonorrheal arthritis, migraine, menopause, etc., and thought it was an excellent antipyretic. A mixture consisting of 0.2 g. acetophenetidin, 0.15 g. phenyldimethylpyrazolone, and 0.05 g. of caffeine was used as an antipyretic in various cases of influenza and colds, usually in doses of two tablets, two or three times a day. These relatively small quantities were quite effective (281). Klein and Kremer (242) describe the use of a mixture of acetophenetidin, 0.4 g., isopropylphenazone, 0.2 g., and caffeine citrate, 0.1 g., and state that the ratio of its toxic dose to its antipyretic dose is 25:1, but they do not present the experimental data. Barthelmes (23) introduced, as an antipyretic for pediatric use, suppositories, each containing 0.1 g. aspirin, 0.1 g. acetophenetidin, 0.005 g. codeine phosphate, 0.0025 g. caffeine, and 0.03 g. phenobarbital. It was effective in reducing the fever of children with a number of diseases including otitis, bronchitis, bronchopneumonia, and cystitis. Wolf (521) used suppositories containing a mixture of drugs, one of which was acetophenetidin, in 50 children, 1 to 13 months old, and found that the antipyretic action began in $^1/_2$ to 3 hours.

During the first few years after its introduction, acetophenetidin received widespread use as an antipyretic. It reduced fever, no matter from what cause, and usually was free of side-effects. It did not cause nausea, vomiting, or depression of the appetite. It had no adverse effects on the circulation, and in reasonable doses it did not produce cyanosis or collapse. Although an active antipyretic in patients with fever, it did not alter the temperature of normal subjects. No contraindications to its use were apparent. Patients with respiratory disturbances or nephritis could take it without demonstrable harmful effects.

N-Acetyl-p-aminophenol. There is at least one early report of the use of *N*-acetyl-*p*-aminophenol as an antipyretic. Hinsberg and Treupel (207) studied its antipyretic action in the human. They found that 0.5 g. of *N*-acetyl-*p*-aminophenol corresponded in its antipyretic action to 0.7 g. of acetophenetidin. Recently there appeared a report (84) of the effectiveness of an elixir of the drug as an antipyretic in children. Colgan and Mintz (79) compared the antipyretic effect of *N*-acetyl-*p*-aminophenol and acetylsalicylic acid in children. They found the maximal effect of each at about 3 hours, with the onset somewhat later and the duration longer after aspirin administration.

Experimental Observations

Chickens. Studies of the antipyretic action of acetophenetidin in experimental animals began quite early. In 1888 Gaiffe (144,145) gave chickens doses up to 2 g. of acetophenetidin per kg. and observed a decrease in temperature of 2°C. Misrachi and Rifat (1888) first gave a 1.0-kg. chicken, 0.2 g. and then 0.05 g. of acetophenetidin and observed no change in temperature, but when they gave 0.11 g. subcutaneously to another chicken the temperature fell from 40.6 to 38.8°C. after 4.5 hours.

Mice. Heubner and Silber (204) described various new antipyretic drugs, and for purposes of comparison acetophenetidin was administered in a dose of 5 mg. per mouse. A fall in temperature from 37 to 33°C. occurred in approximately 2 hours. It returned to normal in 8 or 9 hours.

Pohle and Dittrich (380) studied the antipyretic effect of a combination of acetophenetidin and sulfonal in mice. They found that the mixture had a higher therapeutic ratio as an antipyretic than either alone.

Rats. Gilman and Barbour (155) produced fever in rats by the subcutaneous injection of yeast and compared the antipyretic action of neocinchophen and acetophenetidin alone and in combination. The drugs were administered orally in acacia suspension 18 hours after removal of food. Acetophenetidin in doses of 100 mg. per kg., either alone or in combination with neocinchophen, 250 mg. per kg., produced a maximal effect almost immediately. This was due to the acetophenetidin; the antipyresis due to neocinchophen began later, the effect of the two being almost exactly additive. This is illustrated in Figure 4.

In experiments on rats when artificial fever was produced by the injection of dried yeast (52), the temperature rose slowly to reach a constant level 14 to 16 hours after treatment. Eight of these animals received acetophenetidin, 40 mg. per kg., another group received aspirin, 40 mg. per kg., and still another received an acacia suspension alone. Seven days later the crossover test was done. Later an experiment was performed comparing aspirin, 66 mg. per kg., with acetophenetidin, 40 mg. per kg. Brownlee concluded that acetophenetidin was superior as an antipyretic. In a later study, Brownlee and Gaddum (54) also compared several antipyretic drugs in rats made febrile by the injection of dried yeast. They concluded that for an equal antipyretic effect the following doses of drugs were required in mg. per kg.: acetophenetidin, 40; acetanilid, 24; aminopyrine, 31; and aspirin, 54. Eagle and Carlson (108) produced fever in rats with a suspension of yeast and found that the average maximal fall in temperature caused by 100 mg. per kg. of acetophenetidin was 2.0°C., whereas the fall caused by 100 mg. of aspirin per kg. was 0.95°C. Sandberg (411) gave rats 0.3 millimole per kg. of acetophenetidin by stomach tube and found that the temperature of normal animals was scarcely affected. However in those rats that had fever due to the subcutaneous administration of yeast, according to the method of Smith and Hambourger (451), there was an average temperature fall of 1°C. at the end of 1 hour. The temperature gradually returned to pre-medication levels over the next 5 hours. Lewis (277) compared the antipyretic action of acetophenetidin and two other structurally related drugs. In rats with fever caused by yeast injections, the temperature fell from 39.0°C. to a minimum of 37.8°C. in 4 hours following administration of 100 mg. of acetophenetidin per kg. The temperatures at 2 hours and at 6 hours were

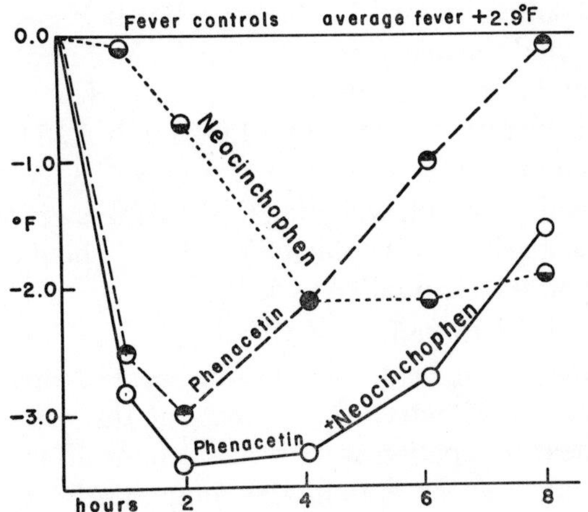

Figure 4. The antipyretic action of acetophenetidin and neocinchophen and their combination in rats. (From Gilman and Barbour, ref. 155.)

about the same. In the control animals the temperature decreased from 38.9 to 38.3°C. in the same 4-hour period.

Boréus and Sandberg (37) studying the antipyretic action of acetophenetidin in female rats in which artificial fever was produced by the injection of a yeast suspension found that barbital and carbromal antagonized the antipyretic effect. The same authors (38) compared the antipyretic action of acetophenetidin and *N*-acetyl-*p*-aminophenol in rats and found both of them to be effective at 50 and 70 mg. per kg.

Noach *et al.* (354) observed that several doses of acetophenetidin produced a decrease in body temperature of adrenalectomized rats but not normal rats. They concluded the adrenals were not necessary for antipyresis.

A mixture of 0.3 millimole per kg. of acetophenetidin and of diallylbarbituric acid produced a marked decrease in the body temperature of normal rats but scarcely more than by the barbiturate alone. When the same mixture was given to rats fevered by yeast injections, the effects were additive, resulting in a marked and prolonged antipyresis (411).

Rabbits. Forschelen (135) gave a rabbit subcutaneously 0.5 g. of an alcoholic solution of acetophenetidin. Some 6.5 hours later the temperature of the rabbit had actually risen 0.4°C. Gaiffe (144,145) gave 2.5 g. acetophenetidin to a 1.5-kg. rabbit and observed a marked decrease in temperature. Éloy (117) discussed these results and those which Gaiffe obtained in chickens, but it is not clear whether or not he repeated the experiments himself. Mahnert (307) gave an 0.87-kg. rabbit 1.5 g. of the drug and noticed that the temperature was lowered 2°C. after 30 min. In a 1.0-kg. rabbit, 3.0 g. of the drug produced a fall in temperature from 39.1 to 31.7°C. with death after 16 hours. Another rabbit, weighing 0.65 kg., was given 4.5 g. of the drug intramuscularly. This animal died after 30 hours, during which time the temperature had fallen to 36°C.

Ott (359) tested the effect of the drug on rabbits, giving it by capsule, and measuring heat reduction and heat dissipation by means of a d'Arsonval calorimeter. The effects of the drug on heat production and heat dissipation were tested 1 hour after its administration. With only one exception, the temperature was reduced in several experiments. Heat dissipation was reduced in 4 out of 6 experiments, and heat production diminished in 5 of 6 experiments.

Garcia y Mansilla (147) gave a rabbit weighing 0.68 kg. an emulsion of 1.5 g. acetophenetidin orally and noticed that the temperature decreased 1.0°C. in 15 min., 1.7°C. in 30 min., and 2.7°C. in 90 min. Two and one-half hours after the drug was given the animal was cold to the touch with a temperature of 34.8°C. One-half hour after this the temperature began to rise until it reached its initial value 5½ hours after the drug had been given. Another rabbit weighing 1.01 kg. was treated similarly and in 20 min. the rectal temperature had dropped to 35.7°C. The body temperature diminished until the animal died 6 hours after administration of the drug; the temperature just before death was 30°C.

Muirhead (344) discussed the mechanism of action of antipyretics but he did not give any original data. He stated that, if the cord of a rabbit were cut below the corpus striatum, the drug failed to reduce fever. If the connection was severed above the corpus striatum, the drug reduced the temperature by decreasing heat dissipation, causing vasodilation and perspiration just as when the nervous system was intact.

Torboli (482) gave 260 mg. of acetophenetidin per kg. and observed a decrease in temperature in rabbits with fever artificially produced of 1.3 to 1.8°C. in about 2.5 hours. Warren and Werner (506) produced fever in rabbits by injection of a pyrogen from *Proteus vulgaris*. Six control animals were employed each test day and six for each dose level of the drug. The average rectal temperature in the animals increased from 39.7 to 41.1°C. with a peak at 4 hours. Acetophenetidin in doses up to and including toxic doses of 800 mg. per kg. decreased the fever but failed to restore the rectal temperatures to normal. However, the elevated temperatures could be reduced to normal or below normal by aminopyrine, acetanilid, or aspirin. According to Bruns *et al.* (55), usually 1500 mg. acetophenetidin per kg. in an oral suspension was ineffective as an antipyretic in rabbits, but occasionally it did produce a temperature fall of 2°C.

When barbital was administered in doses of 20 to 100 mg. per kg. together with acetophenetidin, there was an increased effect; the largest fall in temperature after acetophenetidin alone was 2.5°C., but with barbital added a maximum decrease of 4.7°C. was obtained in 20 out of 30 cases. Bruns *et al.* concluded that the effect of barbital was synergistic, but did not depend closely upon the dose. Urethane also acted synergistically with acetophenetidin. They concluded that the effect of these hypnotics on acetophenetidin antipyresis was nonspecific and that acetophenetidin acted not only on the hypothalamic heat center but also on the entire thermal regulating centers of the central nervous system. Enders *et al.* (118) studied the effect of adding caffeine to antipyretics on their ability to reduce fever in rabbits made febrile by the injection of methylcellulose. He observed less antipyresis when the caffeine was added than when acetophenetidin alone was given. He had no explanation for this, but he did point out that it did not necessarily follow that the analgetic effect of the drug was altered in a similar way by caffeine.

Cats. Brownlee (52) compared the antipyretic activity of acetophenetidin and aspirin after oral administration to cats made febrile by subcutaneous injections of *Escherichia coli* vaccine. In two cats the temperature rise was evident 1 hour after injection, and they were suitable for an antipyretic study in 2 hours with the effect of the vaccine persisting for 24 hours. Using a crossover type of experiment, he demonstrated that the relative doses of aspirin and acetophenetidin needed to produce a comparable antipyretic effect were in the ratio of 5:3. Acetophenetidin in doses of 33 mg. per kg. was comparable to 54 mg. of aspirin per kg. Brownlee and Gaddum (54) concluded that 33 mg. acetophenetidin per kg. produced an antipyretic effect in cats equivalent to 16.5 mg. acetanilid per kg., 25 mg. aminopyrine per kg., or 54 mg. aspirin per kg.

Dogs. Baldi (22) conducted some of the early studies on the effects of acetophenetidin on the temperature of dogs. A dose of 80 mg. per kg. in one dog resulted in a temperature decrease of 1.0°C., and a dose of 175 mg. per kg. in another dog followed by another dose of 114 mg. per kg. produced a fall in temperature of 1.8°C. Cerna and Carter (70), using a calorimeter, obtained evidence that acetophenetidin reduced heat production in dogs but did not increase heat dissipation.

Winter *et al.* (518) undertook experiments to ascertain whether or not the antipyretic effects of acetophenetidin in the dog could be fortified substantially by the simultaneous administration of magnesium oxide. Adult dogs, fasted for two days, with fever induced by hay infusion, were given orally either acetophenetidin or magnesium oxide or a combination of both. With the combination of

200 mg. per kg. of acetophenetidin and 100 mg. per kg. of magnesium oxide the results obtained were quantitatively similar in all animals to those obtained in 8 dogs with doses of 300 mg. per kg. of acetophenetidin alone. Magnesium oxide by itself in doses of 75 to 300 mg. per kg. produced definite antipyresis in 6 of 15 dogs. They concluded that magnesium oxide substantially enhanced the antipyretic action of acetophenetidin, but that the results did not allow them to decide whether this was a matter of synergism or a simple summation of effects.

Lim and Pindell (279) compared the antipyretic action of aspirin, acetophenetidin, *N*-acetyl-*p*-aminophenol, and a mixture of acetophenetidin, aspirin, and caffeine in dogs. They gave a pyrogen intravenously, and used only those animals which responded with a rise of 0.6°C. or more in temperature. The pyrogen alone produced a rise in temperature of 1.0°C. at 160 min. In their tests they gave the drug orally, 30 min. before the pyrogen. Acetophenetidin at a dose of 200 mg. per kg. produced a linear decrease in body temperature of 0.6°C. and successfully suppressed any rise in temperature for 240 min. A dose of 125 mg. per kg. prevented a rise in body temperature for 120 min.; then the body temperature rose 0.8°C. by the end of 240 min.

Human. Traversa (483) obtained evidence, from the increase in volume of the arm and the increase in skin temperature in each of two patients, that acetophenetidin acted as an antipyretic by causing dilation of the peripheral blood vessels. Stern (468) measured the heat rise produced in normal individuals by physical work. This usually was less than 1°C., and after the administration of acetanilid or antipyrine the rise was appreciably less. It may be assumed that this was also true after acetophenetidin administration but it was not given as one of the examples.

Sokolov (455) studied the influence of antipyrine, acetanilid, acetophenetidin, and other drugs on evaporation through the skin in normal and feverish children. In normal children the skin evaporation rate was appreciably lower than in feverish children. The subjects had a significant lowering of the skin evaporation rate after acetophenetidin which was approximately parallel to the body temperatures.

N-Acetyl-p-aminophenol. The effects of very small doses of *N*-acetyl-*p*-aminophenol in guinea pigs with artificial fever produced by the injection of vaccine were studied by Frommel *et al.* (142). They found that a dose of 2.0 mg. of *N*-acetyl-*p*-aminophenol per kg. produced the same effect as a much larger dose of acetophenetidin. They obtained good antipyretic effects with doses of 2, 5, 10, and 25 mg. of *N*-acetyl-*p*-aminophenol per kg. They found that acetophenetidin, 100 mg. per kg., produced an effect one-half as great as that produced by an antipyrine dose of 15 mg. per kg., while a dose of *N*-acetyl-*p*-aminophenol of 2 mg. per kg. was 25 times as effective as antipyrine.

In rabbits some reduction in fever was produced by doses of 20 mg. per kg. of the drug and a maximal average effect was produced by 100 mg. per kg. (393).

Lim and Pindell (280) compared the antipyretic action of sodium acetylsalicylate and *N*-acetyl-*p*-aminophenol in dogs. They gave a pyrogen intravenously and used only those dogs with a rise of 0.6°C. or more in body temperature. The pyrogen produced a rise in temperature which was almost linear for the first 160 min. *N*-acetyl-*p*-aminophenol, in doses of 100 and 200 mg. per kg. given intravenously at the same time as the pyrogen, produced a significant decrease in fever at 120 min.

It has been comparatively easy to demonstrate the antipyretic action of acetophenetidin and *N*-acetyl-*p*-aminophenol in experimental animals and this action actually has been demonstrated in several species. Mixtures containing acetophenetidin or *N*-acetyl-*p*-aminophenol are also effective as antipyretics, and there is some evidence that the ability of acetophenetidin to reduce temperature is markedly enhanced by the simultaneous administration of barbiturates.

Chapter VII

Analgesic Action

Clinical Observations

In many of the earlier studies it was noticed that acetophenetidin was an effective analgesic. A number of investigators in 1888 reported success with acetophenetidin in the treatment of pain. Cattani (68) used doses of 0.2 to 0.5 g. in the pain associated with malaria and tuberculosis. Dujardin-Beaumetz (102–104) observed that it was an effective drug for vague pains and nervous conditions. In making some early observations on its use Georgievsky (151) noted that one of the most remarkable properties of acetophenetidin was its ability to allay pain. In several cases of headache, one of very severe degree with neuralgia of the trigeminal nerve, the pain was relieved in $^{1}/_{2}$ hour. In migraine, especially in women during their menstrual period, it proved to be very useful. It eased the pain in 2 cases of sciatica, and in 3 cases of tabes its effectiveness was really surprising, since in one of these even morphine had been ineffective. Guttmann (168) reported that he had used acetophenetidin for $^{3}/_{4}$ of a year and that it relieved headaches within 30 min. It also was valuable in tabes and rheumatic pain. Henschen (197) used the drug successfully in doses of 0.5 g. as an antipyretic and in 1.0-g. doses as an analgesic in neuralgia. Heusner (205) found that acetophenetidin was of value in neuralgia, in central nervous system inflammation due to nervousness, in migraine, and in sciatica. Holladay (1888–89) had a patient, a young girl with intense facial and visceral neuralgia, who usually had been given morphine for pain. Acetophenetidin, in 0.4-g. doses every 3 hours, produced relief of pain in $^{1}/_{2}$ hour, and although the pain returned in 2 hours, it was not as severe. There was no more neuralgia after the sixth dose. He thought that acetophenetidin effected quicker and more pleasant relief than antipyrine. Hirschfelder (209) believed that the effectiveness of the drug in rheumatism was due to its antipyretic action, since he observed a decrease in pain along with the sweating. The joint swelling decreased after small doses. However, he usually found salicylates the preferred method of therapy in this condition. Acetophenetidin was effective in neuralgia and migraine because of its prompt and prolonged action and because it could be given over a long period of time without serious side-effects. Hoppe (215) successfully treated a 40-year-old woman with migraine with 1.0-g. doses of acetophenetidin. In most cases of headache the pain disappeared in $^1/_2$ to 2 hours with doses of 1.0 to 1.5 g. In one case of sciatica in which acetanilid and antipyrine had been used without success immediate relief was obtained with acetophenetidin. When the pains were due to an organic derangement such as kidney stones there was only a mild effect. Mahnert (307) said that acetophenetidin had a specific effect on polyarthritic rheumatism with a decrease in the swelling of the joints, pain, and fever, and an increase in perspiration. Acetophenetidin was substituted for antipyrine in a patient with trigeminal neuralgia who had been taking increasing amounts of antipyrine without relief. There was such improvement that after 20 doses of 0.5 g. the patient was dismissed with no more pain. Misrachi (336) believed the drug was effective as an analgesic but he used it in too few cases to determine whether or not it was superior to antipyrine. Müller (346) very early found that acetophenetidin was able to combat neurological pain. It usually was necessary to give 0.5 to 0.7 g., and for headache and typical migraine attacks, it was necessary frequently to give 2.0 to 3.0 g. for successful action. Müller (345) found that in 13 out of 23 patients with joint rheumatism the fever stopped immediately, and the joint pains and swelling stopped in 2 to 5 days. In 6 patients there was no effect. Nissim (353) treated a patient with an intra-orbital tumor which caused great pain and found that 1.0 g. in each of three doses was successful in reducing the pain. Ott (358) found that 2 doses of 0.5 g. at intervals of 1 hour usually were sufficient to relieve neuralgia. Pesce (370) found that a dose of 0.5 g. of acetophenetidin usually was sufficient for the relief of neuralgia and headache if the drug was taken at the onset of the disturbance. Rabuske (388) describes exceptionally good results in a woman who was suffering from a severe case of hemicrania. The attacks started every day at awakening and lasted without interruption until evening when they became less severe. After six doses of 0.5 g. acetophenetidin, which were well tolerated, the attacks stopped. Rifat (395) found it effective against pain but inferior to antipyrine for antipyresis. After the oral administration of 2 to 3 g. in 24 hours in 0.5-g. doses, Schivardi (419) observed good relief of pain and better mobility in arthritis not accompanied by fever. Schoffer (423) reported that a 42-year-old patient with right-sided hemicrania, who had taken acetanilid for 6 months with success but then it became ineffective, obtained relief after two doses of acetophenetidin of 1 g. each. The pain relief lasted 2 weeks; then another attack was aborted with 1 g. of acetophenetidin. He also mentions some cases in which relief of pain was not obtained. Schub (424) observed relief of pain in trigeminal neuralgia from 1.0-g. doses of acetophenetidin in the morning and evening, but Faraggi (124) announced complete failure in one case of suborbital neuralgia. Zadok (527) had success in using 0.6 g. per day in patients with periodic headaches.

In 1889 Ayers (18) observed that 1.3 g. of acetophenetidin relieved the pain of dental neuralgia in 40 min. but that the pain returned in 8 hours. Dujardin-Beaumetz (106) advocated the use of acetophenetidin for all forms of pain including neuralgias, migraine, rheumatic pains, muscular rheumatism, acute articular rheumatism, and tabes. Faulkner (125) found that the drug had a sedative effect in neuralgia and sciatica. Horváth (219) observed that acetophenetidin was a good antirheumatic with cessation of pain occurring 3 hours after he had given 3 g. of the drug. Herpes zoster pain stopped after doses of 0.5 to 1.0 g. In a patient with sciatica the pain stopped after 0.5 g., but 3 days later, even three times this dose was no longer effective. Contrary to earlier opinion, Hottenstein (221) found the drug to be effective in a patient with an extensive organic lesion. Pierce (377) observed that acetophenetidin was helpful in relieving the pain and aching of influenza during an epidemic. It also was analgesic in cases of typhoid fever. Specker (461) reported that the drug was particularly effective in neuralgia, and also recommended its use in rheumatoid arthritis where it acted both as an antipyretic and analgesic. Wirz (519) mentioned several cases in which acetophenetidin was very successful in treating migraine, trigeminal pain, and sciatica.

The following year Ayers (19) used acetophenetidin in migraine and neuralgia with relief of pain in 30 to 60 min. Collischonn (80) used the drug in polyarthritis and muscular rheumatism with the usual dose of 0.75 g. to 1.0 g. four times a day. Much later he claimed that the lack of success with acetophenetidin as an antirheumatic could be ascribed to the low dosage which frequently was administered. Sometimes he gave 1 g. in the morning and 2 in the evening. If after 2 to 3 days there was complete pain relief, small doses were continued so that a total of 30 to 60 g. were administered in three weeks. Usually these large doses were so successful that it was not necessary to use salicylates. Espinosa (121) conducted clinical trials in which he substituted acetophenetidin for antipyrine which he said had been known to cause collapse in typhus patients. He used the drug with success in 25 cases. Garcia y Mansilla (147) observed that when given to a patient suffering from neuralgia it relieved the pain in 1/2 hour and promoted drowsiness. Twombly (490) found that acetophenetidin relieved pain more promptly than acetanilid.

Acetophenetidin, in a dose of 0.3 g. every four hours, provided prompt relief of headache and fever during the first stage of influenza (196). Conkling (83) found it effective for the pain of pneumonia and pleurisy. Paterson (367) observed that doses of 0.3 to 0.6 g. were useful in neuralgia of the fifth nerve. Eldridge (115) gave typhoid fever patients 0.5 g. of acetophenetidin and obtained great relief from the pain of the severe headaches. He also observed (116) relief of fever and pain in a four-year-old girl with malaria. Cmuchal (77) used the drug in 0.5-g. doses as an antipyretic and analgesic in several cases.

Warner (505) said that acetophenetidin was less potent than opium as an analgesic but that it did not disturb the stomach and intestinal tract. It was too feeble a remedy to use in peritonitis, pleurisy, or brain tumors, and did not compare with opium in these cases. It relieved neuralgia and sciatica more effectively than acetanilid or antipyrine, but it was of no value in intestinal disturbances where antispasmodics were indicated.

Acetophenetidin-Containing Mixtures. It will be remembered that acetophenetidin was introduced at a time when polypharmacy flourished, and soon the drug was included in various mixtures used for the relief of pain. The other drugs in the mixtures were various, most including the common analgesics such as acetanilid, acetylsalicylic acid, antipyrine, barbital, dihydromorphinone, phenobarbital, phenyl salicylate, and quinine.

Pierce (377) used acetophenetidin in combination with an equal amount of phenyl salicylate in the treatment of rheumatism and influenza. Haller (174) found that this identical mixture of drugs in doses of 0.15 g. was quite effective in relieving the pain in 314 cases of influenza.

Tingley (480) observed a young married woman subject to migraine who could take acetophenetidin without ill effects. However, if she took champagne along with it, even after an interval of hours, her face became flushed, the conjunctival vessels dilated and assumed a bright reddish color, and the face became mottled in appearance. These symptoms usually occurred 20 min. to 1/2 hour after taking champagne and were produced only by champagne or other sparkling wines. This was said to have occurred in 3 patients all of whom could take acetophenetidin alone or with whiskey, brandy, or claret without discomfort. Robertson (399) deplored the routine use of antipyretics but recommended giving whiskey at the same time to prevent untoward effects.

Garrano (148) used a mixture of 4 g. of phenetsal and 1 g. of acetophenetidin in four doses in the treatment of 2 cases of hemicrania. It was successful over a period of many weeks without any side-effects. Treupel (487) mentioned the great advantage that could be gained by administering acetophenetidin, aspirin, and codeine in combination. He believed this to be of special value in cases of inflammation which produced pain and restlessness. He said that in such a combination both the acetophenetidin and codeine acted as analgesics and that healing was promoted through the immobilization of the joints produced by the sedation. In considering the relative merits of the antipyretic drugs and opiates, Sajous (409) observed that 0.25 g. of acetophenetidin was an effective analgesic dose. Von Noorden (355) and Loewe (287) considered the advantages in the use of mixtures of barbital, acetophenetidin, and codeine. Waegner (501) discussed a mixture of 0.15 g. of acetophenetidin, 0.1 g. of phenylquinolinic acid, and 0.075 g. of calcium citrate which he used for a number of clinical conditions and which he claimed to be without side-effects. Collischonn (81) described the use of pastilles containing acetophenetidin in the treatment of diseases of the mouth and pharynx. He thought that in simple inflammation of the mouth there was sufficient absorption perlingually of the acetophenetidin and other compounds to produce marked analgesia. Markovics (314) discusses a mixture containing codeine,

0.01 g., acetophenetidin, 0.25 g., and aspirin, 0.25 g. He used it in 50 to 60 gynecological cases including dysmenorrhea, and found it to be such an effective analgesic that he used it to replace morphine partially. This same mixture in suppository form, each containing codeine phosphate, 0.02 g., aspirin, 0.5 g., and acetophenetidin, 0.5 g., is reported by Schulze (425) to be promptly effective in post-tonsillectomy patients and in patients with inflammation and infections of the inner ear. Martin and Blumentritt (315) believed a mixture containing 0.2 g. acetophenetidin, 0.1 g. barbital, and 5 mg. of papaverine was of value in the therapy of headache, migraine, and neuralgia, because the papaverine relaxed the musculature so that the aspirin and barbiturate might work more effectively. Dressen (100) said that a mixture containing codeine phosphate, aspirin, and acetophenetidin was an effective analgesic, without side-effects, for adults in doses of 2 tablets three times a day. Trepte (485) used a mixture containing codeine phosphate, 0.01 g., aspirin, 0.25 g., acetophenetidin, 0.25 g., quinine, 0.03 g., and magnesia, 0.06 g., in doses of 2 tablets in tabes, neuralgia, and dysmenorrhea. Busch (60) used a mixture of caffeine, 0.05 g., and 0.15 g. each of acetophenetidin, phenyldimethylpyrazine, and dimethylaminophenazone in approximately 100 cases of gonorrheal arthritis, migraine, and menopause, and noticed that smaller doses of morphine and barbital were then required. Nesnera (351) considered a mixture of 0.3 g. each of quinine, acetophenetidin, and aspirin to be quite effective in 1500 cases of influenza. A mixture consisting of 0.2 g. acetophenetidin, 0.15 g. phenyldimethylpyrazolone and 0.05 g. caffeine was found to be particularly good for headaches, neuralgia, and trigeminal pain and for the after effects of alcohol, nicotine, and X-rays (281); three tablets were believed to be almost as effective an analgesic as a dose of morphine. Waggoner (502), in discussing the choice of analgesics, recommended for severe pain a mixture of aspirin, 0.23 g., acetophenetidin, 0.17 g., caffeine, 0.03 g., and codeine sulfate, 0.017 g. Ainlay (2) found a mixture of aspirin, 0.3 g., acetophenetidin, 0.2 g., and propadrine hydrochloride, 0.05 g., to be effective for dysmenorrhea. Maloney (310), endeavoring to evolve a combination of dilaudid in which its effectiveness was unimpaired while its undesirable side-effects were suppressed, used a mixture of acetophenetidin, acetanilid, and dilaudid, as well as a combination of dilaudid, acetophenetidin, and a barbiturate. Both mixtures were effective in treating the common cold.

Another study in patients with acute upper respiratory infections was conducted by McLane (322). One group of the patients received tablets containing 0.5 g. aspirin, 0.12 g. acetophenetidin, and 0.03 g. caffeine. Another group received this same mixture plus 0.025 g. phenyltoloxamine dihydrogen citrate, while a third group received the four-component mixture plus 100,000 units of procaine penicillin G. All patients took two tablets of the preparation three times a day for a total of 16 tablets. When observed after 72 hours only 2 per cent of the group receiving the mixture containing penicillin had failed to improve, while 53 per cent and 46 per cent, respectively, of the first two groups had failed to show improvement. Bergstermann *et al.* (29) used a mixture of 0.2 g. salicylamide, 0.2 g. acetophenetidin, 0.03 g. caffeine, and 0.02 g. benzyl benzoate for the therapy of headaches and dysmenorrhea. He believed it was more effective than aspirin. In 78 cases of dysmenorrhea, 56 patients reported complete relief of pain. Lüdecke (292) observed 60 patients with acute or chronic rheumatoid myasthenia, rheumatoid arthritis, neuralgia, sciatica, influenza, or herpes zoster over a period of 6 months. He administered a mixture of salicylamide, acetophenetidin, caffeine citrate, and phenylquinoline carboxylic acid for a week or more. Excellent analgesia was obtained in all the disorders except rheumatoid arthritis. In 1953 Rabenalt (387) claimed that a mixture containing papaverine, phenobarbital, caffeine, dimethylaminophenazone, and acetophenetidin combined the central action of phenobarbital, the spasmolytic action of papaverine, and the analgesic action of dimethylaminophenazone and acetophenetidin. He believed that the caffeine increased the total effect. This combination was particularly useful in goiter operations and in headaches localized in the neck and rear of the head. Usually its action lasted 3 to 4 hours. Ordinarily it was employed no longer than 8 or 10 days because the symptoms were no longer present.

Klein and Kremer (242) used a mixture of 0.4 g. acetophenetidin, 0.2 g. isopropylphenazone, and 0.1 g. caffeine citrate in 93 gynecological patients and observed excellent analgesia in postpartum women. McLane and Heck (323) studied the effect of a mixture of 0.12 g. acetophenetidin, 0.15 g. aspirin, and 0.03 g. caffeine along with antihistamines and penicillin in upper respiratory infections.

Two tablets were given three times a day and the responses evaluated after 72 hours. The mixture containing penicillin gave a much better response in most of the patients. A mixture of acetophenetidin, 0.17 g., aspirin, 0.17 g., amobarbital, 0.03 g., and *d*-amphetamine sulfate, 5 mg., produced 83.5 per cent relief of moderate pain in 50 patients, and Hanes (179) believed it to be slightly superior in this respect to an ordinary mixture of acetophenetidin, aspirin, and caffeine. There was a definite mood elevation in most patients, although a few complained of insomnia. Ottoson (361) found that a mixture consisting of acetophenetidin, dibenzyl aminoethanol chloride, phenemal, and caffeine was as effective as an analgesic in post-tonsillectomy patients who were given 1 tablet three times a day. A mixture of caffeine, phenyldimethylpyrazolone, acetophenetidin, and lactylphenetidin was observed by Seiler (431) to be a fast acting and effective analgesic in dental patients.

Five reports have appeared (35,140,141,408,508) attesting to the value in the therapy of headaches of a mixture, each tablet containing 130 mg. acetophenetidin, 200 mg. aspirin, 40 mg. caffeine, and 50 mg. isobutylallylbarbituric acid.

Recently Völker (479) gave one group of patients 6 to 8 tablets a day, each containing 0.1 g. phenyldimethylpyrazolone, 0.1 g. quinine hydrochloride, and 0.05 g. ascorbic acid for the treatment of respiratory infections. He believed that the results were somewhat better than those in another group given 400,000 units of penicillin only.

Harris and Bird (184) conducted a double-blind study in a home for chronic patients and the aged. Altogether there were 437 separate treatments in 25 patients, who were given either 2 tablets of 0.3 g. aspirin or 2 tablets each containing 0.194 g. aspirin, 0.13 g. acetophenetidin, and 0.022 g. caffeine plus aluminum hydroxide and magnesium hydroxide. Pain relief with the mixture was 81.1 per cent compared with 75 per cent with aspirin alone. The authors believed that the relief actually was greater and faster with the mixture and that it produced slightly fewer side-effects. More recently Wittich (520) and Pagano (363) report success in the therapy of vascular headaches and migraine through the use of a mixture containing 130 mg. acetophenetidin, 100 mg. caffeine, 1.0 mg. ergotamine tartrate, and 0.1 mg. belladonna alkaloids. Presumably the same mixture was studied by Cass *et al.* (67) who found that it compared favorably with a buffered aspirin preparation as an analgesic.

Pagano (364), in a study of patients with migraine, said that acetophenetidin exerts "its analgesic action on the residual pain in the occipital area caused by sustained contractions of the skeletal muscles of the head and neck."

Holtzem (214) reported favorable results in the therapy of rheumatic fever with a mixture containing acetophenetidin.

It is common to find that investigators who have studied the treatment of headache with many drugs conclude, as do Friedman and Merritt (139), that "The most practical and useful analgesics used in the treatment of headaches are the antipyretic coal-tar derivatives, such as acetylsalicylic acid and acetophenetidin." It is interesting that the two drugs acetophenetidin and aspirin, are used so frequently in analgesic mixtures. Speaking of this, Krantz and Carr (255) state, "the two analgesics in smaller doses appear to be more effective in relieving pain in a greater number of people than either drug alone in its full analgesic dose. There is no adequate pharmacologic explanation for this observation."

N-Acetyl-p-aminophenol. Batterman and Grossman (25) obtained better analgesia in patients with musculo-skeletal pain with *N*-acetyl-*p*-aminophenol than with acetylsalicylic acid. They obtained satisfactory analgesia in 66 per cent of 234 patients with acetophenetidin and in 5 per cent with aspirin. An elixir containing 120 mg. *N*-acetyl-*p*-aminophenol has been reported to be an effective analgesic in children (84). In chronic rheumatism it compared favorably as an analgesic with codeine compound tablets, and there were fewer side-effects (177).

Soon after acetophenetidin came to be so widely used as an antipyretic, it became evident that it was also an effective analgesic drug. It was recognized early to be an effective remedy in migraine, sciatica, dental neuralgia, trigeminal pain, and rheumatoid arthritis. While successful against the pain and discomfort associated with typhoid fever, tuberculosis, and influenza, it was soon appreciated that it had no specific effect upon the infection.

Experimental Observations in Animals

Mice. Hesse (198) used as an analgesic test the pinching of the tails of mice with an artery clamp. Acetophenetidin in doses of 1300 mg. per kg. was analgesic in 4 out of 6 animals, and 1500 mg. per kg. was analgesic in 6 out of 10. Pohle and Dittrich (380) found that

700 mg. of acetophenetidin per kg. was analgesic in mice. The same information was given in later reports by Pohle and Vogel (382) and Pohle and Spieckermann (381). In analgesic experiments in mice in which pain was produced by attaching an arterial clamp to the tail and to the anal mucosa, Hesse and Kuegler (200) observed that acetophenetidin, aminopyrine, and certain other drugs were effective in reducing the pain. Siegmund *et al.* (435) injected phenylquinone intraperitoneally into mice and induced "writhing, presumably associated with pain." The condition responded immediately to the oral administration of 260 mg. acetophenetidin per kg. The peak effect was at 30 min. as it was after doses of 165 mg. aspirin per kg. (436).

Ogiu *et al.* (357) gave 20 mice 0.2 g. acetophenetidin per kg. intraperitoneally plus 5 mg. morphine per kg. subcutaneously and observed some evidence of analgesia in 4 animals. Pohle and Dittrich (380) found that a mixture of acetophenetidin and sulfonal in mice was less toxic and less analgesic than acetophenetidin alone. A mixture of acetophenetidin and urethane in mice had a higher therapeutic ratio than acetophenetidin alone (382), as did a mixture of acetophenetidin and barbital (381).

N-Acetyl-*p*-aminophenol, given intraperitoneally to mice (334) in doses of 629 to 818 mg. per kg., produced analgesia.

Rats. Sivadjian (438) reviewed briefly the various methods used to determine analgesic action. His own method consisted of a cage with electrical wires at the bottom on which the rat rested. The current required to produce a shock with a painful reaction was defined as the minimal stimulus. Morphine produced an increase in the pain threshold but no increase was observed with acetophenetidin and several other drugs including salicylates. Macht and Macht (302) induced pain by faradic stimulation of the adult male rat scrotum. In the unanesthetized rat, the stimulus caused the rat to squeal and also caused the cremasteric muscle and muscle fiber of dartos tissue to contract. Using 30 mg. of acetophenetidin, presumably the total dose, the voltage necessary initially was 155; after 45 min. it was 265; after 2 hours it was 250. Comparable data with aspirin in 30-mg. doses were 135, 140, and 120 volts; and with the same amount of aminopyrine, 250, 265, and 809 volts. Smith *et al.* (439) used a method adapated from that of Hardy and Wolff by determining the intensity of light required to cause a rat to flick its tail. No analgesia was produced by the nonopiate drugs unless the dose was very large. Acetophenetidin was given subcutaneously at a level of 600 mg. per kg. without any analgesia being observed. When it was given orally in doses of 700 mg. per kg. and 900 mg. per kg. slight analgesia was produced.

Hart (189) modified the analgetic method devised by D'Amour and Smith by arranging the apparatus so that the animal was exposed to a warmth stimulus before the pain stimulus was applied. The amount of drug necessary to produce significant analgesia in 50 per cent of a group of animals, using 15 or more animals at each dose, was 0.56 g. of acetophenetidin per kg., 0.18 g. acetanilid per kg., and 0.35 g. aspirin per kg. In a similar study Renault *et al.* (393) observed that a moderate increase in the time required to produce a response was produced by 0.5 g. acetophenetidin per kg.

Eagle and Carlson (108) used a method employing an algesimeter for measuring subcutaneous pain threshold in rats. The minimal stimulus capable of evoking a response was determined in triplicate for each rat, just before and at hourly intervals after drug administration. Using 200 mg. of acetophenetidin per kg. in 20 rats, the highest average algesimetric value was 61 compared with 21 in the case of comparable doses of aspirin. La Belle and Tornaben (260) used rats that had been injected in the ankle joint with silver nitrate. No evidence of analgesic effect was obtained during a period of 24 hours after the oral administration of the drug in doses of 1000 mg. per kg., although the swelling was reduced significantly, as it also was after a comparable dose of aspirin. Boréus and Sandberg (37) found a significant effect with 50 and 70 mg. acetophenetidin per kg. in 1 hour; this diminished in the next 2 hours. Lewis (277) compared certain properties of acetophenetidin and two closely related drugs with respect to the pain threshold of rats measured by the radiation thermal stimulation method. The mean reaction time after 100 mg. of acetophenetidin per kg. given intraperitoneally was increased from 3.2 to 3.6 sec. It was increased from 3.0 to 3.8 sec. after 200 mg. per kg., and it was increased from 3.1 to 4.4 sec. after 400 mg. per kg.

Gibson *et al.* (153) published a method for the evaluation of nonnarcotic analgesics which depends upon the squeak response of rats to graded electrical stimuli, using a contact rectal electrode. The drugs were given orally in 10 per cent acacia. They found that the analgesic activity of salicylates seemed to be parallel with the blood salicylate levels. The minimal effective oral doses and relative analgesic potencies of the other drugs were compared with those of acetylsalicylic acid. Acetophenetidin in a dose of 750 mg. per kg. was 0.6 as effective as acetylsalicylic acid in a dose of 450 mg. per kg.

Smith *et al.* (439) studied the analgesic properties of certain drug combinations with respect to the pain produced by a beam of light focused on the tip of a rat's tail. When acetophenetidin was given subcutaneously, no analgesia was produced with a 600 mg. per kg. dose, or with a mixture of acetanilid, 300 mg. per kg., plus acetophenetidin, 300 mg. per kg., but a significant analgesia was obtained with a mixture of aspirin, 300 mg. per kg., plus acetophenetidin, 300 mg. per kg. However, when they gave orally aspirin, 500 mg. per kg., plus acetophenetidin, 450 mg. per kg., only slight analgesia was produced and none at all was obtained with a mixture of acetophenetidin, 450 mg. per kg., plus aspirin, 500 mg. per kg., or with a combination of acetanilid, aminopyrine, and acetophenetidin, 225 mg. per kg. of each. Sandberg (412) observed that the analgesic action of acetophenetidin in rats was augmented by the simultaneous administration of 5,5-diallylbarbituric acid. There also was synergism of the analgetic action. Boréus and Sandberg (37,39) used a modification of the Ercoli and Lewis (119) technique, which in turn was a modification of the Wolff, Hardy, and Goodell (522) technique, in which radiant heat was applied to the shaved backs of rats and the rapid twitching of the skin was observed as an indication of a response. They found that acetophenetidin alone was a better analgesic than a mixture of it with barbital. Barbital and carbromal both antagonized not only its analgesic action but its antipyretic action as well.

Gibson *et al.* (153), using rats stimulated by a graded electrical shock through a contact rectal electrode, found that the following mixtures all were appreciably less effective than acetophenetidin alone in a dose of 750 mg. per kg.: 150 mg. aspirin plus 100 mg. acetophenetidin per kg.; 150 mg. aspirin plus 110 mg. acetophenetidin plus 22 mg. caffeine per kg.; and 300 mg. aspirin plus 220 mg. acetophenetidin plus 44 mg. caffeine per kg. A mixture of 300 mg. aspirin plus 220 mg. acetophenetidin per kg. was approximately as effective or perhaps slightly more effective than 750 mg. acetophenetidin per kg. by itself.

N-Acetyl-p-aminophenol. In doses of 50 mg. per kg. and 70 mg. per kg., *N*-acetyl-*p*-aminophenol, given to rats by stomach tube, produced a significant analgesic effect in 1 hour which then diminished in the next 2 hours (37). The same authors, Boréus and Sandberg, in a later paper (38) determined the analgesic effect of this compound on rats, using the modifications of the Ercoli-Lewis technique, and did observe an analgesic effect with 200 mg. per kg. given orally. They found a slightly higher analgesic action with 200 mg. acetophenetidin per kg. than with the same dose of *N*-acetyl-*p*-aminophenol but the difference was not statistically significant. Other investigators (332) found that 57 mg. of *N*-acetyl-*p*-aminophenol per kg. was analgesic in rats, producing a slightly higher elevation in threshold than that produced by a placebo of saline given intraperitoneally in a similar way. Their method of producing pain was by the application of a hot wire to the tail of the rat. *N*-acetyl-*p*-aminophenol in doses of 2025 to 3037 mg. per kg. produced analgesia and hypnosis (334).

Guinea pigs. Haffner (169) compared in guinea pigs several analgesic drugs by measuring the pressure which it was necessary to exert on a clamp on the ear of the animals in order to produce a vocal response. Acetophenetidin was effective at 3000 mg. per kg. whereas aminopyrine was effective at 150 mg. per kg. Hesse *et al.* (202) used guinea pigs injected with croton oil and, measuring the pressure required to produce pain at the site of inflammation, observed no analgesia with 800 mg. acetophenetidin per kg.

Rabbits. Fleisch and Dolivo (132) reported a definite increase in the stimulant threshold determined by stimulating the tooth pulp after the animals were given 100 mg. or 300 mg. of acetophenetidin per kg. orally. The results are illustrated in Figure 5. Frommel *et al.* (142), using an electrical shock method in rabbits, found that 200 mg. of acetophenetidin per kg. gave about a 50 per cent elevation of analgesic threshold at about 75 min. whereas 200 mg. of aminopyrine per kg. produced a 100 per cent elevation.

N-Acetyl-*p*-aminophenol, in a dose of 50 mg. per kg., gave about a 10 per cent elevation of pain threshold (142).

Cats. Albright (4) used the method of Eddy (110) which involved putting a weight on the tail of a cat and found that acetophenetidin and one other drug were the weakest of the substances tried.

Dogs. Espinosa (121) injected subcutaneously a dog weighing 2.5 kg. the first day with 1 g. acetophenetidin, the second day with 0.25 g., and the third day with 0.5 g. The dog did not exhibit signs of pain when pricked with a pin. The animal returned to normal 2 hours after the last dose.

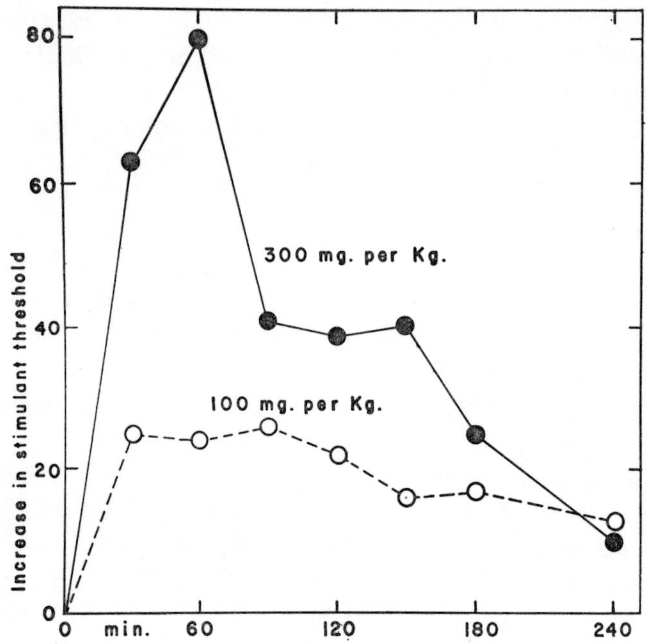

Figure 5. The increase in stimulant threshold for the tooth pulp of the rabbit after acetophenetidin. (From Fleisch and Dolivo, ref. 132.)

In summarizing much of the data Goetzl (157) said that the results of animal experiments showed that at least 13 tests in mice could be interpreted as indicating that the drug was able to raise the pain threshold. (These results were obtained partly by means of mechanical and partly by means of electrical methods.) Some of the results of the remaining tests on various animals had to be interpreted as indicating that the drug was not effective, while still others did not permit either conclusion with certainty.

As with all of the drugs of the analgesic type, other than the narcotic drugs, it is difficult to assess activity in experimental animals. Recently Beecher (26) has presented detailed criticisms of the many methods used to assess analgesic action in experimental animals and concluded that while the techniques have definite usefulness in predicting the effectiveness of the powerful narcotics, apparently they are of little value with the milder analgesics. The available evidence indicates that acetophenetidin compares favorably with the other drugs of this group. There are fewer studies on *N*-acetyl-*p*-aminophenol but these indicate that it too is an effective analgetic drug.

Experimental Observations in Patients and Normal Human Subjects

Much time and effort have gone into devising adequate methods for demonstrating experimentally in the human the analgesic action of acetophenetidin and related drugs. Although their effectiveness is well recognized, it has been difficult to evaluate this experimentally and no procedure has gained wide acceptance. The experimental techniques for studying pain in man have been criticized by Beecher (26). He concludes that all of them probably are useless for the appraisal of analgesic agents.

Martin *et al.* (316) studied the changes in electro-cutaneous sensitivity produced by various analgesic drugs. Two of the authors determined each other's sensory threshold initially and again an hour later. The drug was taken in 0.3, 0.6, and 1.0 g. doses in gelatin capsules immediately after the first set of readings. The experimental period was limited to 1 hour. Fourteen control tests were made, 7 on each subject. In the control readings, neither subject showed variations which exceeded 10 per cent in either direction. They did, however, show a marked difference in initial sensitivity. One subject took a 0.3-g. dose three times and showed an average increase of about 40 per cent in the stimulus required to produce cutaneous sensation. When the same subject was given 0.6 g. on two occasions the average change was about 23 per cent. When the subject was given 1.0 g. on six occasions the average change was about 16 per cent. The other subject took the 0.3-g. dose three times and obtained, respectively, increases of 28 per cent and 20 per cent, and a decrease of 9 per cent. He took the 0.6-g. dose six times with an average increase of about 20 per cent. He took the 1.0-g. dose three times for an average change of about 30 per cent. Hale and Grabfield (172) used the same subcutaneous threshold method and, after giving doses varying from 0.2 to 0.5 g., determined the threshold at 30-min. intervals for 90 min. after the drug was taken. The effect of acetophenetidin with a maximum in $^1/_2$ hour was more prolonged than that of antipyrine. Aspirin had no effect on the threshold.

Hesse and Reichelt (201) did a comparative study in human subjects using electrical stimulation of the tooth pulp of healthy and of carious individuals. The authors concluded that acetophenetidin was an effective analgesic in the human. Ebbinghaus (109), using the electrical pain threshold of teeth, found that acetophenetidin, in a dose of 0.5 g., produced a maximal effect in 20 min., which lasted for 30 min., the total duration of action being 72 min. Vollrath (498) used the tooth pulp method and found that 0.5 g. acetophenetidin reached its maximal action after 70 min., and aspirin after 30 min. The effect of acetophenetidin disappeared in 2 hours and that of aspirin in 1 hour. Contrary to other authors, notably Münchau (349), Strohschnieder (470) used the tooth pulp method and found that of the four analgesics tested in doses of 1 g., acetophenetidin was the weakest and also had the shortest duration of action. The strongest and longest acting was aspirin. The effect, however, was produced more rapidly with acetophenetidin than with the other drugs, the maximum being reached after 30 min.

Wolff *et al.* (522), also Hardy *et al.* (181), determined individual pain thresholds by focusing the light from a 1000-watt lamp on the blackened forehead of a subject. Control tests were repeated every 30 to 60 sec. until the patient felt pain at the end of the exposure period of 3 sec. After analgesics were given, observations were made at 10 to 20 min. intervals until these returned to the control level. Sleep was not allowed. Two experiments with 0.3 g. of acetophenetidin, representing six series of observations, were made. The results are illustrated in Figure 6.

Burrill *et al.* (59) compared the analgesic action of several well-known drugs to amphetamine, using dental students and applying an electric current to teeth fillings. The same tooth and filling were used in all tests for any one subject. Drugs were administered and readings taken every $^1/_2$ hour for 2 hours. A 0.4-g. dose of acetophenetidin produced a voltage threshold rise in 10 subjects, a fall in 4, and no change in 3. When 0.5 g. was given along with 5 mg. *dl*-amphetamine, there was a rise in 10, a fall in 3, and no change in 3. Placebos alone gave a rise in 42 subjects, a fall in 51, and no change in 25.

Goetzl *et al.* (158) studied the analgesic effect of acetophenetidin in human subjects. Goetzl (157) summarized some of the results obtained using the tooth pulp method, and observed that while in 38 tests there was a rise of threshold, there was none in 31 of the

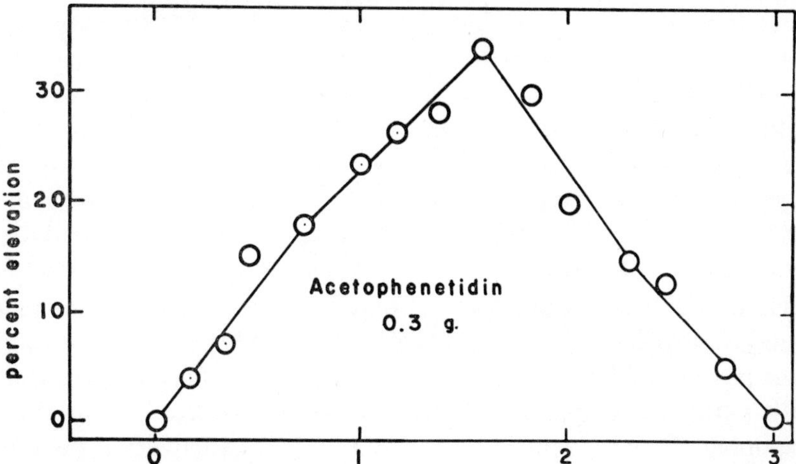

Figure 6. The average pain threshold elevation resulting from the administration of 0.3 g. acetophenetidin to normal human subjects. (From Wolff *et al.*, ref. 522.)

tests. The results in the remaining 54 tests did not permit either interpretation with certainty. In all of the thermal tests there was a rise in pain threshold. There were no essential differences between aspirin, acetophenetidin, and aminopyrine regarding their pain threshold raising action when administered in doses of 0.3 g. With the electrical method of inducing pain, the threshold was raised by aspirin in 11 per cent of the experiments, by acetophenetidin in 31 per cent, and by aminopyrine in 50 per cent. There was no rise in threshold in 65 per cent of the experiments with aspirin, 25 per cent with acetophenetidin, and 33 per cent with aminopyrine. Sonnenschein and Ivy (459) used the tooth pulp method of Goetzl *et al.* in 20 subjects. In no case was there a significant rise in tooth pulp threshold with any of the doses of acetophenetidin up to 1.95 g. nor was there any with the usual dose of aspirin. From these results they concluded that "It is reasonable to suppose that they counteract the pathological processes which produce pain secondarily in both headache and arthritis."

Acetophenetidin-Containing Mixtures. Hale and Grabfield (1923) investigated the effect of smoking on the threshold of sensation for an electric current applied to the skin. There were striking effects with both acetophenetidin and antipyrine. Instead of the usual increase in irritability of 2 or 3 per cent at the end of the first 1/2 hour, they found with antipyrine an average fall of irritability of 30 per cent, provided the subjects were not smoking. In the smoking experiments the fall was reduced to 5 per cent. With acetophenetidin the rise in threshold was more continuous and prolonged, reaching a maximum 90 min. after ingestion. In smoking experiments the initial effect could be traced but the curve of irritability returned to within normal limits after the first 1/2 hour. It was evident that smoking antagonized the effect of these drugs upon the threshold.

Heinroth (195), using stimulation of tooth pulp to produce pain, found that when 0.5 g. of acetophenetidin plus 0.2 g. caffeine sodium benzoate were given orally, there was a decrease in pain sensitivity with a peak at 80 min. and a return to normal after 3 hours. When acetophenetidin was mixed with barbital there was very little additional change in the pain threshold. Wesemann (511) used the tooth pulp method and found that 0.5 g. of acetophenetidin was the optimal dose to produce analgesia. If more was given he obtained a smaller effect. The optimal dose for diallylbarbituric acid was 0.1 g. When the two drugs were combined there was an additive effect as may be seen in Figure 7. Münchau (349) found by the tooth pulp test that the effect of caffeine in increasing the intensity of analgesia was insignificant but there was a slight lengthening of the time of analgesia. Vollrath (498) using the tooth pulp method found that in humans acetophenetidin reached its peak of action at 70 min. in doses of 0.5 g. and that two mixtures of acetophenetidin, either with aspirin or with codeine, were more effective than acetophenetidin alone. Wolff *et al.* (522) found that a combination of 0.3 g. each of acetophenetidin, acetanilid, and aspirin had no greater effect than 0.9 g. of aspirin alone; however, the sedative and hypnotic effects of the combination were far greater than those of the aspirin alone. When the acetophenetidin was given by itself there was a 35 per cent increase in threshold in about 2 hours. The threshold returned to normal after 3 hours.

Harris and Brandel (185) used the tooth pulp stimulation method for their studies of 14 subjects who received each of the following

4 test regimens: codeine phosphate, 0.065 g., a mixture of 0.3 g. aspirin plus 0.3 g. acetophenetidin, calcium lactate placebos, nothing at all. The drugs were put up in identical appearing capsules. They concluded that the demonstrable analgesic effects of the mixture of aspirin and acetophenetidin were better than those of the placebos. Harris and Worley (186) compared the pain threshold

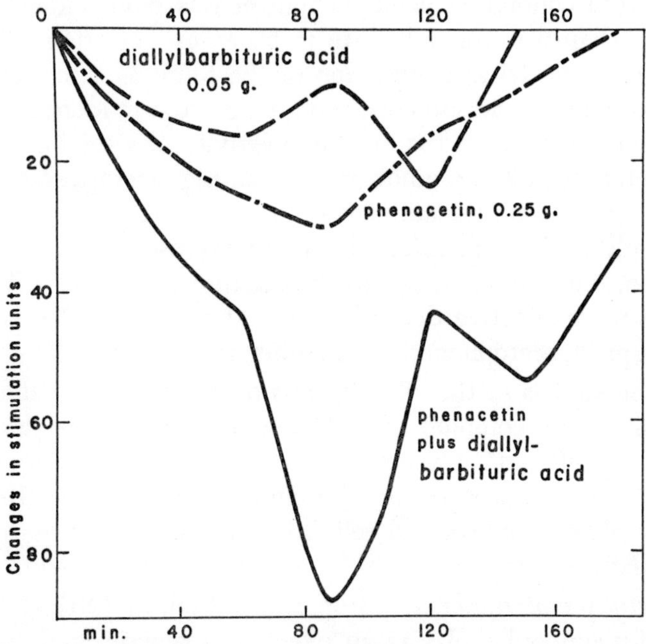

Figure 7. The analgesic effect of acetophenetidin, of a barbiturate, and of their combination in human subjects. (From Wesemann, ref. 511.)

elevating capacity of a mixture of 5 mg. *d*-amphetamine sulfate, 32 mg. amobarbital, 162 mg. aspirin, and 162 mg. acetophenetidin with a mixture composed solely of the same dose of aspirin plus acetophenetidin. They determined the electrical threshold of pain in the tooth pulp three times at 15-min. intervals before medication. The mixture of aspirin and acetophenetidin did not produce a statistically significant effect. There was a good effect when the four-component mixture was given.

Hoffmann (210) produced pain in human subjects by a sphygmomanometer cuff on the arm and studied various combinations of acetophenetidin with salicylamide and aspirin. One compound contained acetophenetidin, salicylamide, aminopyrine, and caffeine.

The specific analgesic effects of acetophenetidin were not separated from those of the other drugs. Davies (91) compared the analgesic effect in patients of 0.65 g. of 1-phenyl-2,3-dimethyl-4-methylamino-pyrazalone-*N*-methane sulfonate with a mixture of 0.52 g. aspirin, 0.52 g. acetophenetidin, and 0.016 g. codeine phosphate. He reported that 15 per cent of the patients obtained relief with placebos. The mixture containing acetophenetidin was more effective as an analgesic than was the sulfonate in 59 cases. Harris and Worley (187), using electrical stimulation of the tooth as a means of producing pain in normal subjects, and giving drugs in identical appearing capsules, compared the analgetic activity of a mixture of 5 mg. *d*-amphetamine, 32 mg. amobarbital, 162 mg. acetophenetidin, and 162 mg. aspirin with the activity of some other drugs. Observations were made at 20-min. intervals after administration. In patients with pain, 9 out of 10 preferred the mixture to codeine. This mixture was more effective than placebos, 30 mg. of codeine, or a mixture of aspirin, acetophenetidin, caffeine, and codeine.

In some studies of the effectiveness of citrus bioflavonoids in the treatment of the common cold, Macon (303) gave, as the control drug, 16 capsules, in 2 days, of a mixture, each capsule containing 1.3 gr. aspirin, 1.0 gr. acetophenetidin, and 0.2 gr. caffeine. He attributed complete or substantial relief, in more than half the patients, to the mixture.

N-Acetyl-p-aminophenol. Brodie and Axelrod (45) stated that *N*-acetyl-*p*-aminophenol was an effective analgesic, and in a later study Flinn and Brodie (133) used a modification of the cutaneous heat-radiation method on 12 trained human female subjects. Duplicate control measurements were within 3 per cent. The threshold to pain rose within 30 min. following the administration of 0.2 g. of drug. The peak action was reached in 2.5 hours, and the threshold returned to normal in about 4 hours. The maximal rise in pain threshold above the control level averaged 30 per cent, while that with a placebo averaged 4 per cent. They concluded that the analgesic action of *N*-acetyl-*p*-aminophenol in a therapeutic dose is comparable to that of acetanilid in the same dose. Wallenstein and Houde (503), in a double-blind test in 27 cancer patients, compared the analgesic action of 0.6 g. *N*-acetyl-*p*-aminophenol with that of 0.6 g. salicylamide, 0.6 g. aspirin, or a lactose placebo. They measured the "relief scores" for up to 6 hours. The time curves for aspirin and *N*-acetyl-*p*-aminophenol were quite similar and were higher than those for salicylamide or lactose. The probability that the effect was due to chance was less than 1 in 100. Houde (222) compared the analgesic action of identical capsules containing either of the following: 0.36 g. aspirin, a mixture of 0.21 g. aspirin plus 0.15 g. *N*-acetyl-*p*-aminophenol, and 0.03 g. caffeine, or 0.36 g. *N*-acetyl-*p*-aminophenol alone. In a preliminary report he found that the drug combinations were better than any one drug alone. The caffeine contributed nothing to their effectiveness.

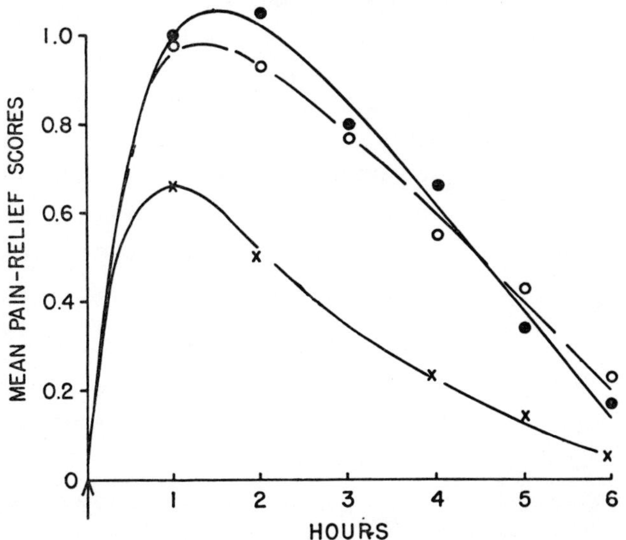

Figure 8. Comparative analgesic effect in patients of *N*-acetyl-*p*-aminophenol and aspirin. x = placebo; • = 0.6 g. aspirin; o = 0.6 g. *N*-acetyl-*p*-aminophenol. (From Houde, ref. 222.)

Boréus *et al.* (40) observed the relief of pain after dental surgery by the administration of several mixtures containing *N*-acetyl-*p*-aminophenol, salicylamide, and one or more of the following ingredients: amobarbital, diallylbarbituric acid, codeine phosphate, and caffeine. In general all the mixtures were effective analgesics.

In an exceptionally well-controlled study, Newton and Tanner (352), using a double-blind test in arthritis patients, compared the analgesic action of 1.0-g. doses of *N*-acetyl-*p*-aminophenol with a mixture containing 0.52 g. acetophenetidin, 0.52 g. aspirin, and 0.016 g. codeine. Although the method of sequential analysis revealed that the codeine compound tablets on the average were superior as an analgesic, some patients regularly preferred *N*-acetyl-*p*-aminophenol, and there were consistent side-effects in only 3 patients, all of them receiving codeine compound. Their conclusion that there is a consistent preference of *N*-acetyl-*p*-aminophenol by some patients has been questioned by Hajnal (170).

Most of the evidence indicates that acetophenetidin is an effective analgesic when tested experimentally in human subjects. Some data indicate that the drug may be effective in relieving the pain peripherally. The small amount of data on *N*-acetyl-*p*-aminophenol in human subjects indicate that it is as effective as acetophenetidin.

Few drugs enjoy such wide use as analgesics clinically and in home medication. There is a wealth of data supporting the value of acetophenetidin as an analgesic. Its effectiveness in headache, post-traumatic pain of tooth extraction, and generalized aches and pains of muscle and joint origin cannot be denied.

Chapter VIII

Other Therapeutic Uses

Clinical Observations

Very early several authors noted the effectiveness of acetophenetidin in articular rheumatism. Müller (345) reports that in 13 of 23 patients with rheumatism the joint pains and swelling stopped within 2 to 5 days. Mahnert (308) found that acetophenetidin had a specific effect in polyarthritic rheumatism in addition to its antipyretic effect, causing a decrease in pain, fever, and the swelling of joints. Schivardi (419) observed good relief of pain and better mobility in arthritis patients without fever. Price (386) also noted that in acute rheumatism of the elbows, wrists, knees, and ankles the drug produced reduction of swelling with return of the use of the joints. Rifat (397) observed considerable relief in cases of rheumatoid arthritis when patients were given 3.0 g. of the drug on the first day followed by 5.0 g. each day for 3 days.

There are early reports of the use of acetophenetidin as a dusting powder. Eldridge (116) used the drug locally for ulcers. Lee (268) describes several cases in which he applied the drug as a finely powdered substance to the ulcerated portions of wounds. In an injury with a rip saw, the wound did not heal readily until after he began to use acetophenetidin locally.

Probably because of the early success with acetophenetidin as an antipyretic, some investigators (8) attributed success to the use of the drug in certain infectious diseases. For instance it was mentioned that 60 cases of typhoid fever, when treated in this way, resulted in but 1 fatality and this occurred in a patient who had not received acetophenetidin until 3 weeks after the beginning of the attack. There were no complications in any of the other cases. Pel (368) stated that the drug was not curative in infections and did not have a specific chemotherapeutic action. Michaelis (329) found that antipyrine had no effect in whooping cough, but acetophenetidin was quite effective. One patient with whooping cough had 15 attacks of coughing a day before using the drug; this was reduced to

3 with acetophenetidin and on some days there were no attacks at all (194). When drug administration was stopped, the attacks occurred with their previous frequency and severity.

Heusner (205) used acetophenetidin against insomnia and found it to be very effective. He advised administering it in alcohol because of the increased solubility of the drug but did not mention that the solvent might have contributed to the hypnotic effect. Klemperer (243) thought that a mixture of 4 parts of acetophenetidin and 2 parts of barbital produced a desirable sedation in mental patients. Wolff *et al.* (522) called attention to the relaxation and drowsiness produced by acetophenetidin. There also was slight impairment of concentration, retention, and attention. Restlessness was allayed and anxiety was diminished, but there was no euphoria.

Using a mixture of which 2 tablets contained 0.3 g. sodium barbital, 0.25 g. acetophenetidin, and 0.025 g. of codeine phosphate, Baer (21) estimated that the mixture decreased by about one-half the necessary dose of barbiturate necessary for hypnosis and sedation. Mönkemöller (338) found that 2 tablets each containing 0.3 g. sodium barbital, 0.25 g. acetophenetidin, and 0.025 g. codeine phosphate were effective as a hypnotic and sedative in psychiatric patients. Von Noorden (355) used the identical mixture and found that it had the same hypnotic effect as 0.6 g. barbital. A mixture of diphenhydramine, 50 mg., caffeine, 200 mg., acetophenetidin, 250 mg., and codeine, 30 mg., was found to be a useful hypnotic in elderly patients (134). A mixture, each tablet of which contained 0.10 g. acetophenetidin and 0.25 g. salicylamide, produced adequate sedation in 77 per cent of 157 persons with insomnia not due to pain (43). There were few side-reactions and no evidence of allergy or intolerance. Of 54 patients previously requiring a hypnotic, 79 per cent responded to the mixture. Lendon (270) has suggested that, since the salicylates in themselves have little power to induce sleep, manufacturers add acetophenetidin, codeine, etc. to make the mixtures more universally useful.

Trebing (484) used tablets containing 0.3 g. sodium barbital, 0.25 g. acetophenetidin, and 0.025 g. codeine phosphate and found that he could substitute them for morphine as pre-anesthesia medication to the use of ether. He found that there was little effect if the drug was given immediately before the ether but he obtained an optimal response when the mixture was given 1.5 hours prior to the ether.

He observed that less ether was required during the operation and that less nausea and vomiting occurred afterwards.

Albrecht (3) found that suppositories containing 0.1 g. aspirin, 0.1 g. acetophenetidin, 0.005 g. codeine phosphate, 0.0025 g. anhydrous caffeine, and 0.03 g. phenobarbital were effective in quieting children afflicted with bronchial pneumonia and pertussis.

In a controlled study of the effects of several drugs in the treatment of nonspecific respiratory infections, Cronk *et al.* (90) found no significant difference between a group treated with a mixture containing 0.16 g. aspirin, 0.13 g. acetophenetidin, and 0.03 g. caffeine and similar groups given the same drugs plus phenyltoloxamine diacetate, procaine penicillin, and salicylamide. Aside from the use of acetophenetidin as an analgesic in upper respiratory infections there is some evidence that its use in mixtures diminishes the duration of illness in influenza. Rosenberger (404) distributed tablets, each containing 0.1 g. aspirin, 0.1 g. acetophenetidin, 0.05 g. ascorbic acid, and 0.01 g. quinine hydrochloride to 3000 workers in an industrial plant. They were instructed to take 1 or 2 tablets three times a day if they felt any symptoms of influenza infection. The sickness rate during a season reckoned critical for an influenza epidemic was approximately 6 per cent, compared with about twice this in neighboring factories, and the duration of illness was diminished.

When 30 patients each were given 4 tablets each containing 0.2 g. acetophenetidin and 0.03 g. of caffeine, each day for 3 successive days, their symptoms of hay-fever were not reduced more than in those patients given a placebo control. Lowenstein (290) observed that this mixture produced prompt relief of the symptoms of seasickness. It was used for seasickness also by von Noorden.

Seitz (432) has used a mixture containing 0.5 g. acetophenetidin and 0.05 g. codeine phosphate and found it to be useful in the treatment of disturbed urination on a functional basis.

Experimental Observations

Stender (467) studied the potentiation of the local anesthetic properties of cocaine and its various derivatives by acetophenetidin using the cornea of the guinea pig eye. A 0.15 per cent solution of cocaine had a weak local anesthetic effect which was potentiated appreciably by acetophenetidin, as well as by aminopyrine and antipyrine. The local anesthetic action of β-eucaine also was potentiated by acetophenetidin. Acetophenetidin was inferior however to antipyrine and lactophenine in this respect.

Acetophenetidin prolonged the hypnotic action of barbital in mice in which the doses of acetophenetidin varied from 0.1 to 1.0 g. per kg. and of barbital from 0.05 to 0.2 g. per kg. (199). In a study of sedative action (277), acetophenetidin was injected intraperitoneally in mice 30 min. before a standard hypnotic dose of 100 mg. hexabarbital sodium per kg. The control mice received only the barbiturate. The geometric mean sleeping times of the groups of control animals and of those receiving various doses of acetophenetidin were determined and the per cent increase over the control calculated. A dose of 114 mg. acetophenetidin per kg. was necessary to increase the duration of hexobarbital hypnosis 50 per cent. Groups of rats receiving acetophenetidin in combination with 1.0 mg. *d*-desoxyephedrine hydrochloride per kg. were compared with groups receiving *d*-desoxyephedrine alone, in order to determine the extent to which the first drug could antagonize the stimulating action of the second. The acetophenetidin was given orally while the *d*-desoxyephedrine was given subcutaneously. With a dose of 200 mg. of acetophenetidin there was no reduction in stimulation caused by the *d*-desoxyephedrine.

It may be recalled that acetophenetidin was introduced as an antipyretic at a time when it was believed that all antipyretics had some antiseptic or bactericidal action. Müller (345) found that acetophenetidin might delay the growth of some microorganisms, and that it inhibited the formation of red pigment by *Micrococcus prodigiosus*. This pigment was formed normally when the white culture was reinoculated on a new peptone-gelatin medium. Müller (347) mentioned that acetophenetidin had little antiseptic properties and thus there was no necessary parallelism between antiseptic and antipyretic effects. Garcia y Mansilla (147) mixed a drop of putrified liquid obtained from prolonged maceration of fresh greens with a hot solution of acetophenetidin. When observed under the microscope the infusoria and bacteria moved freely, even after 24 hours, so he concluded that the drug had no antiseptic properties. Duca *et al.* (101), in studies on the chemotherapy of tuberculosis, concluded that acetophenetidin did not possess any significant *in vitro* activity against the organisms. More than 32 mg. per cent was required to inhibit each of two strains of tubercle bacilli.

In a study on animals with spontaneous tumors (489), 10 mice of the C_3H strain were given 5.0 mg. of acetophenetidin per dose intraperitoneally. Such mice lived 23 days and their tumors regressed 1.0 to 5.0 mm. as compared with control mice which lived 57 days and in which the tumors grew 18 mm. When 10 mice of the SWR strain were given daily doses of 1.87 mg. of acetophenetidin intraperitoneally, the mice lived 77 days and the tumors grew 9 mm., whereas the control animals lived 48 days and the tumors grew 12 mm. This indicates that with a larger dose of 5.0 mg. of acetophenetidin equivalent to about 250 mg. per kg. per dose, the life span of the mice was shortened and the tumor regressed slightly, perhaps due to the toxic effects of the drug.

There is no convincing data that acetophenetidin is effective against experimental tumors to any extent greater than might be expected from the administration of large doses of many other agents.

Using tissue cultures consisting of pieces of monkey testicular tissue, Kramer *et al.* demonstrated (254,447) that acetophenetidin had a very slight inhibitory effect on the type 2 poliomyelitis virus at the relatively large concentration of 4.0 mg. per ml.

N-Acetyl-*p*-aminophenol, tested against poliomyelitis virus in explants of monkey testicular tissue (254,448), was inhibitory at a concentration of 2.5 mg. per ml. and showed evidence of toxicity at a dose of 10.0 mg. per ml.

Chapter IX

Effects on Blood and Organ Systems

Central Effects

Clinical Observations

In an early description of the effects of acetophenetidin, Köbler (245) observed that a majority of the patients who used the drug as an antipyretic became euphoric. They felt at ease while the more spontaneous among them became talkative and had an increase in appetite.

Rumpf (406) mentioned that he did not notice the euphoria described by Köbler; on the other hand, Forschelen (135) did observe euphoria in some of his patients. Very often they became more talkative and their appetite increased.

Illoway (225) attended an 18-year-old obese girl who had suffered from amenorrhea for several months. She went home from work with a severe headache and took 1 powder containing 0.3 g. of acetophenetidin. A few hours later she had a violent convulsion, with the spasms recurring at short intervals. However, he learned later that this girl had had convulsions some years previously. In another case, 9 days after the birth of her third child, a 30-year-old woman had a severe headache and fever for which 0.3 g. of acetophenetidin and 0.06 g. caffeine were prescribed. Shortly afterward she was seized with severe typical hystero-epileptic convulsions which were followed by two further seizures of equal severity in rapid succession. There was no recurrence after this and she recovered in 6 weeks after having suffered from mental depression and melancholia. He gave no details as to the earlier history of this patient.

Hoppe (215) observed tinnitus once or twice after acetophenetidin administration. It was noticed especially in patients who had been weakened by disease, and the role of the drug in its production is not established. One was a woman with leukemia having a high temperature. She was given 0.2 g. of the drug and developed a tinnitus by the following day. A 48-year-old workman with fever took 0.7 g. of acetophenetidin every 2 hours for a total of 7 g. (167) and developed deafness though the eardrums were intact. Meningitis was ruled out but he was reported to have had pneumonia and herpes from chin to eyes. The deafness persisted for 6 days. After 5 months the patient returned to work but was said to have impaired hearing. Although the author concluded that the deafness was caused by acetophenetidin, this may be questioned in light of the extensive herpes of the face. A 32-year-old male with caries and trigeminal neuralgia developed a tachycardia, decrease of hearing ability, intense heat with profuse sweating, nausea, and vomiting some hours after the third dose of acetophenetidin (114). After vomiting the symptoms completely disappeared. The patient felt extremely well. He took 1 g. of acetophenetidin on another morning and none of these symptoms was observed. Fernández de Ybarra (128,129) reported that a woman with intense headaches took 1.3 g. of acetophenetidin and in a few minutes was in convulsions, but she was out of danger in 1 hour. There was no mention of whether she had been subject to previous convulsive seizures.

Poljakov (383) describes a student who took 60 g. of acetophenetidin and complained of dizziness, his consciousness was dim, he was apathetic, and responded unwillingly. The pupils were enlarged and reactive and the reflexes were intact. Later his condition became worse and he began to convulse. The next day he still had occasional convulsions.

Hamill and Hine (176) described a 37-year-old woman suffering from chronic colitis who had been treated with paratyphoid vaccine prepared from organisms recovered from her stools. The day after her third injection of vaccine and after taking an unknown number of 0.3-g. acetophenetidin tablets, her mind wandered and she became delirious. Intervals of lucidity or of restlessness, alternated with periods in which she was semicomatose. It seems reasonable to ascribe the deliriousness to the high fever induced. Fisher (131) mentioned a 47-year-old man who took large amounts of acetanilid and acetophenetidin over a long period of time, usually as much as 8 g. of acetanilid and 3 g. of acetophenetidin daily. There were marked mental symptoms after the drugs were discontinued. The patient became confused and irrational and developed ideas of reference and persecution. These symptoms gradually disappeared in the course of a week or two. There was no record that the patient was emotionally stable prior to observation by the physician and no reason is given for his taking the excessive doses.

Schweingruber (426) reported that in 40 cases with untoward effects attributed to acetophenetidin, 28 per cent had some central nervous system symptoms. It is not clear whether these existed prior to acetophenetidin ingestion or were attributed by the author to the drug.

Experimental Observations

Frogs. Godelbarrer (156) studied the depressant action of acetophenetidin on tadpoles. In a 0.0025 molar solution of acetophenetidin, the reflexes were lost in 10 min. but were recovered in spring water after 10 min. In a 0.0012 molar solution, the reflexes were lost in 20 min. and recovered in 2. Using frogs which had been given large doses of acetophenetidin, Hare (182) tied off the artery supplying the left leg of the animals to protect it from the effects of the circulating drug. Since he found that there was still a failure of reflex activity in the leg, he concluded that the effect was on the cord.

Mice. Berger (28) found that acetophenetidin had no true hypnotic action in mice. It failed to produce loss of righting reflexes when it was given in doses appreciably below those that were fatal. Mixtures of equal parts of acetophenetidin and salicylamide or of one part acetophenetidin and three parts salicylamide were effective and safe hypnotics in mice. There was no hypnosis when acetophenetidin was given with acetamide, *p*-phthalamide, 2-furamide, nicotinamide, gentisamide, salicylate, gentisate, aspirin, salol, *p*-aminobenzoic acid, *p*-acetylaminophenylsalicylate, antipyrine, aminopyrine, or pyribenzamine.

Rats. Ubaldi (491,492) observed that when rodents were given large doses of acetophenetidin they developed tetanic convulsions.

Acetophenetidin in doses of 4 or 5 mg., as well as acetanilid and aminopyrine, depressed the activity of rats in a circular maze (296). Acetanilid and acetophenetidin appeared to be a depressant mixture for rats. A mixture of acetophenetidin plus aminopyrine produced less depression.

Doses of 25 mg. of magnesium phenobarbital plus 124 mg. of acetophenetidin per kg. produced excitement and slight hypnosis in rats whereas double this amount produced a depression lasting several hours (154). A combination of acetophenetidin and phenobarbital was appreciably less toxic than phenobarbital alone. On the other hand, aspirin also antagonized the hypnotic action of phenobarbital.

Sandberg (412) gave rats 0.3 millimoles of acetophenetidin or of diallylbarbituric acid or of a mixture of the two. He found that acetophenetidin did not influence the duration of the anesthetic action of the barbiturate but that the two drugs were additive in their analgesic effects. Doses of 200 mg. of acetophenetidin per kg., given by mouth to rats treated with 1.0 mg. of *d*-desoxyephedrine hydrochloride subcutaneously, did not antagonize the stimulant action of the desoxyephedrine (277).

Guinea pigs. Hinsberg and Treupel (207) gave a 461-g. guinea pig, 1.5 g. of the drug orally. After 90 min. it had a clonic convulsion and appeared to be half asleep.

Rabbits. Mahnert (308) noticed that 3 g. of acetophenetidin in a 1-kg. rabbit produced disturbances in equilibrium. Garcia y Mansilla (147) gave orally 3 g. of acetophenetidin to a 1-kg. rabbit, and 10 min. later the animal had convulsions. Tainter *et al.* (476) used an electrical device for measuring the convulsive threshold of unanesthetized rabbits. Acetophenetidin raised the convulsive threshold as did acetanilid, but only in very high doses. With acetophenetidin depression was demonstrable but the doses required were so high compared to those clinically effective that the authors concluded that the therapeutically useful action does not depend upon the type of change measured in these experiments.

Dogs. A 2.5-kg. dog given 2.5 g. of the drug had convulsions after a few minutes, first clonic and then tonic, resembling those seen after strychnine poisoning (121). The same effect was produced in two other dogs. Large doses were observed by Ledoux (267) to produce convulsions. He also observed intense salivation.

Falcone and Gioffredi (122) reported nervous system lesions produced by the prolonged use of acetophenetidin, presumably in the dog, although the animal used was not specified. They mentioned destruction of the spinocerebellar paths with resulting incoordination of movements as well as lesions of the Purkinje cell, but they gave no details of their experiments.

Masetti (318) gave the drug orally to a dog and increased the dose gradually until after 2½ months a daily dose of 3.5 g. was reached. At the beginning of the third month of the experiment, the animal lost its natural liveliness, the walk became rigid, unstable, and staggering. It crossed its legs, especially its hind ones when it walked, and seemed to be in extreme fatigue. The pupils remained normal to light stimuli. He said that the drug acted upon the central nervous system, and in toxic doses affected the cerebral nerves creating degenerative recessive processes. He concluded that these effects could be produced only after the prolonged use of very large doses.

Human. Using two healthy young medical students, Martin *et al.* (316) studied the effect of acetophenetidin upon electro-cutaneous sensitivity. The drug was taken in 0.3-, 0.7-, and 1.0-g. doses in gelatin capsules. In control studies without the drug one subject showed a rise in threshold and the other a fall, but the variation did not exceed 10 per cent in either direction. After giving acetophenetidin there was a definite loss in sensitivity.

In studies of the influence of various drugs on the neuromuscular coordination test of "tapping," Macht *et al.* (299) used 0.3 g. alone and in combination with acetanilid, 0.3 g., or phenyl salicylate, 0.3 g. Acetophenetidin showed a definite tendency to improve the tapping rate as did acetanilid, antipyrine, aspirin, and quinine. The results were not striking. Doses exceeding 0.5 g. tended to impair efficiency of performance.

The reaction time was measured in subjects after doses of 0.3 g. of several analgesic drugs (301). Acetophenetidin alone and acetophenetidin plus phenyl salicylate produced either very little change in reaction time or impaired it slightly. The simple reactions to sound, light, and touch were more affected than complex reaction times.

Macht *et al.* (300) also studied the effect of some of these drugs on the field of vision. Acetanilid, acetophenetidin, and aspirin in doses of 0.3 g. produced a definite though not marked increase in the visual field, especially in the case of white and blue.

Acetophenetidin, in doses of 0.17 g. and 0.3 g. was found to improve hearing, and phenyl salicylate distinctly impaired it (297). A combination of the two, however, produced an improvement of 66 per cent over the normal.

Later Macht *et al.* (298) studied the effects of acetophenetidin on normal human subjects and subjects with mild deafness. The drugs were given orally, and the hearing tested before and after at definite time intervals. He stated that acetanilid, aspirin, and phenyl salicylate decreased the acuity of hearing and that antipyrine, aminopyrine, and small doses of quinine increased acuity. Acetophenetidin also was given in therapeutic doses, but the author does not mention the outcome of the experiments.

The effects of acetophenetidin on the sensory threshold for faradic stimulation in human subjects and the influence on this of tobacco smoking were studied by Hale and Grabfield (173). After acetophenetidin, they observed a fairly continuous and prolonged rise in irritability, but smoking brought the curve of irritability to within normal limits after the first $^1/_2$ hour.

Gregg (164) tested the ability of normal human subjects to feel a stimulus applied by a controlled electric vibrator. The vibrator was placed over a test spot on the right quadriceps area. Placebos were found not to produce any change. One of the drugs given was acetophenetidin in doses of 1 g., and observations were made every 10 min. for 120 min. after its administration. In 54 per cent of the cases the subjects did not feel the vibration until the amplitude had been increased. Fourteen per cent of the subjects detected a decrease in vibratory threshold, and 24 per cent found no change. This compared with 59 per cent of the subjects who had diminished response to the vibrations after 1 g. of aspirin, 11 per cent who had an increased response, and 23 per cent who had no change. The maximal effect was observed about 30 min. after ingestion of the drug. He also studied the effects of a mixture of acetophenetidin and aspirin and of aspirin, acetophenetidin, and caffeine.

Roback *et al.* (398) studied the flicker-fusion threshold in 12 normal white male subjects, aged 20 to 34 years, some of whom were given 0.2 g. of *N*-acetyl-*p*-aminophenol in combination with other drugs. All of the drugs and drug combinations depressed the flicker-fusion frequency with a maximum depression at 30 to 90 min. and recovery at 120 min. It is not possible from the data presented to determine the effects either of acetophenetidin or of *N*-acetyl-*p*-aminophenol alone.

Povorinskii (385) has reported some of the effects of acetophenetidin upon the central nervous system.

N-Acetyl-p-aminophenol. Mice and rats, when given very large doses of *N*-acetyl-*p*-aminophenol became sleepy with ataxia and tremors (334). The doses required were appreciably greater than the LD_{50}.

Whereas in experimental animals, very large doses of acetophenetidin exert a depressant effect beyond that associated with analgesia and antipyresis, there is insufficient evidence that in the human the drug has any other significant central depressant effects, such as hypnosis, euphoria, loss of hearing, or elevation of convulsive threshold. Even in large doses it has little tendency to produce nausea or vomiting. Symptoms of tinnitus or of vertigo are rare and ordinarily do not occur even after relatively large doses. There is less evidence concerning the effects of *N*-acetyl-*p*-aminophenol, but the data available do not indicate any significant central depressant effects.

Cardiovascular System

Clinical Observations

Early clinicians using the drug did not note that acetophenetidin had any effect on the contraction of the heart. For instance Mahnert (308) mentioned that it had no effect on the contraction of the heart of children given ordinary doses. Cesari and Burani (72) observed that acetophenetidin was well tolerated by the circulatory system.

As is to be expected, there were some reports in which the possibility of cardiac derangement was mentioned. Fernández de Ybarra (128,129) noted that a woman suffered from convulsions and strong cardiac pain after taking several doses of the drug. She had been drinking beer the night before and had a severe headache. When a 32-year-old woman with dysmenorrhea took 3.3 to 5.3 g. of acetophenetidin in 24 hours, she had a rapid pulse and palpitation of the heart, and her face was scarlet (10). West (512) noted that repeated large doses lowered the blood pressure and sometimes produced evidence of feeble heart action. Knowles (244) reported the case of a 30-year-old woman with a severe attack of migraine who took 2 headache powders and later 0.6 g. of acetophenetidin and suffered near collapse with a pulse of only 40 per min. especially perceptible at the wrist. However, when heat was applied and she was given digitalis, nux vomica, and brandy she began to improve immediately and in 3 hours felt well again. Brunton (56) reported that acetophenetidin, in common with the other antipyretics, had the power of depressing the heart and believed it to be dangerous in large doses. He believed that it lowered the temperature so quickly that it took away stimulus given to the heart by warm circulating blood.

In a report by Laurence (265), a woman over 40 years of age, feeling feverish, was sent by her physician to the drug store for 10 gr. each of acetophenetidin and antikamnia. Through error the prescription was filled for 10 g. of each, and she took at one dose an estimated 5 g. of each. The patient immediately vomited and after several hours felt so ill that she called the druggist to check the dosage. When seen by her physician the heart and respiration were hardly affected, and the patient was soon restored.

Storozhevoj (469) observed a 16-year-old girl who took 25 g. of acetophenetidin. When she was admitted to the hospital her pulse was 100 per min. and weak but regular. The heart had a presystolic murmur that was quite noticeable. He did not record whether this finding persisted after recovery. In 1926 the statement was made (12) that aniline had a direct toxic effect on the heart muscle and that acetophenetidin and other aniline derivatives might bring about symptoms similar to those of aniline poisoning; however, no experimental data were given. Reid (390) reported the case of a 28-year-old woman who was admitted to the hospital with blueness of the lips and fingertips. Her heart was palpable in the fifth interspace at the left mid-clavicular line. The left border of deep cardiac dullness was at the nipple line. The percussion outline of the heart was within normal limits. The action was regular with a rate from 80 to 86 and there were no murmurs, although the heart sounds were softer than usual. The pulse was of a small volume and tension. The blood pressure was 110 systolic, 65 diastolic. An electrocardiogram revealed normal rhythm with a P-R interval of 0.16 second, a QRS interval of 0.06 second, T3 slightly inverted and the axis normal. All waves were of a rather low voltage. Fifteen days later, when she had no evidence of acetophenetidin effects, the heart was the same as before except that its rate was 60 instead of 89. There was no change in the electrocardiogram.

Sears (429) reports a case involving the immoderate use of a mixture of aspirin, acetophenetidin, and caffeine over a 6-year period. The patient took 35 to 50, 5-gr. tablets daily, which provided 8 to 12 g. of aspirin, 5 to 8 g. of acetophenetidin, and 1 to 1.5 g. of caffeine a day. He had a systolic blood pressure of 125 mm. Hg and a diastolic pressure of 80. The heart findings were consistent with heart block; the frequency of the beat was 30 per min. with regular rhythm. After a week without the drug, his pulse was 60 per min. and edema was reduced. The patient obtained the mixture again, became dyspneic, and the pulse rate increased to 180 beats per min. for 12 days. Tachycardia was attended by exhaustion, so an infusion of digitalis was given. The pulse rate fell to 80 in 36 hours and he was clinically improved but died suddenly without a struggle. At autopsy the extensive, generalized atherosclerosis and secondary cardiac changes could not be attributed to the excessive use of drugs. The pathological findings were not traced to excessive use of drugs.

Ainlay (2) used a combination of 0.3 g. aspirin, 0.2 g. acetophenetidin, and 50 mg. of propadrine hydrochloride in 34 cases of primary dysmenorrhea. He usually gave 3 capsules daily until the 3rd day. The blood pressure, taken at intervals over a period of $1^1/_2$ hours after the oral administration of one capsule, showed an average rise of 4 mm. Hg, the peak being reached at the end of 60 min. It dropped to normal at the end of 90 min.

Experimental Observations

Frogs. A frog which had received 8 mg. of acetophenetidin showed a slowing of the heart to 9 or 10 instead of the usual 20 beats per min., but the strength, energy, and regularity of the rhythm did not seem changed (267). When acetophenetidin, 0.04 to 0.07 per cent, was perfused through the hind limb of frogs, there was obvious expansion of the blood vessels (247). The vessels returned to normal when Ringer's solution was substituted for the acetophenetidin solution. Paredes and Lopez (366) perfused isolated frog hearts according to the Straub technique. Acetophenetidin acted on the tone of the myocardium in concentrations of 1:5000 and 1:100, producing a notable elevation. The amplitude of contraction diminished, starting at dilutions of 1:100 or less. These actions were more marked with higher concentrations, which eventually produced diastolic arrest of the heart.

Mice. Kondo (247) reported an expansion of the blood vessels in mice, after perfusing with acetophenetidin, similar to that observed in frogs.

Guinea pigs. When Ledoux (267) gave large doses intravenously to mice, guinea pigs, rabbits, and dogs some effects on the heart were observed. The rhythm and rate of cardiac pulsations were markedly modified. When the drug reached the endocardium there was slowing, but the heart gradually and progressively recovered its force without, however, reaching the same blood pressure as before.

There was an increase in cardiac rate to compensate. The rate of injection was not stated. Hinsberg and Treupel (207) gave a guinea pig weighing 461 g., 1.5 g. of the drug orally. The animal died after about 12 hours, and at autopsy the left ventricle was contracted and the right ventricle filled with blood.

Rabbits. Ott (359) gave a rabbit 0.3 g. of acetophenetidin by mouth, and 1 hour and 20 min. after its administration observed that the pulse rate was unchanged and the blood pressure had fallen by 10 mm. Hg from its initial value of 120 mm. Two min. later the pressure rose 16 mm. but 22 min. after this it had fallen back to its previous level. Garcia y Mansilla (147) gave a rabbit weighing 1.01 kg., 3 g. of acetophenetidin by stomach tube, and about 6 hours later the animal died. At autopsy the heart was in systole and filled with coagulated blood. Similar findings were observed in a rabbit weighing 650 g. which had been given 4 g. of acetophenetidin (6100 mg. per kg.).

Cats. Lagutin (263) studied the effects of the drug on the blood pressure of cats and rabbits, giving the acetophenetidin intravenously. Doses of 9 to 21 mg. into the veins of cats weighing 1 kg. each produced no striking effects on blood pressure. Experiments on 20 cats and 17 rabbits under ether anesthesia, and on 17 rabbits under urethane anesthesia showed that the decrease of blood pressure was greatest 10 to 15 sec. after drug administration, after which it returned to normal. The average lowering of the blood pressure was between 22 and 60 mm. Hg. When the blood pressure returned to normal, a decrease in heart rate was noticeable. On repeated injections of the same doses at 5- to 10-min. intervals there was a noticeable increase in depressive effects, but with injections at intervals of 20 to 30 min. the decrease in blood pressure was more or less uniform. In 6 experiments on isolated cat hearts, Lagutin observed that acetophenetidin in a concentration of 1:4000 produced no changes in rhythm. In a concentration of 1:10,000 acetophenetidin produced a slight diminution in amplitude. In 17 experiments on cats under ether anesthesia, with oncometers on the kidney and back leg, he observed that, with the lowering of the blood pressure, there was a sharp decrease in the size of the kidney and a gradual increase in the dimensions of the leg; then a decrease in the size of the leg was noticeable, which passed very quickly. In cats, after removal of the stomach and intestine, the drug produced an increase in size of the leg and a decrease in the size of the kidney just as before. In an attempt to clarify the effect of acetophenetidin upon the peripheral vessels, Lagutin perfused the drug in concentrations of 1:1000 to 1:4000 into the vessels of isolated ears of rabbits. In all 11 experiments acetophenetidin caused a variable degree of dilation of the vessels. He concluded that dilation of skin vessels was a very important factor in the depressant effect of acetophenetidin on the blood pressure. In order to study the reflex effects upon blood vessel size, experiments were performed on rabbits pretreated either by removing totally the carotid sinuses or by cutting through the sinus nerves. These measures did not have any effect on the intensity of the depressant action. Also the exclusion of reflexes of the cardio-aortic zone to depressor nerves by the complete paralysis of the nerve ends with atropine did not have any effect on the nature and strength of the depressor effect in cats.

Dogs. Baldi (22) studied the effects of acetophenetidin upon the circulatory system of dogs. Traversa (483) observed the effects of acetophenetidin upon the blood vessels of 2 dogs. Ledoux (267) found that acetophenetidin in relatively large doses of 0.25 to 0.5 g. per kg. given intravenously to dogs exerted a long-lasting, depressing influence on the blood pressure. The rhythm and rate were modified appreciably. In early experiments Cerna and Carter (70) found that in a 9.9-kg. dog, the blood pressure remained normal at least for 39 min. after the animal had been given 7 intravenous doses of a 2 per cent suspension of acetophenetidin (10 to 40 ml. each dose) at intervals of 1 to 11 minutes. When a 5 per cent suspension was given to a 20-kg. dog, the first injection of 10 ml. produced a fall in blood pressure followed by recovery in 5 min. The third injection of 10 ml. produced a fall in blood pressure from which the dog recovered in 3 min. Two other doses of 20 ml. caused a progressive fall. When they gave a 28-kg. dog, 1.0-g. doses intravenously, they observed a fall in blood pressure after the fifth dose which continued gradually until death. When a 5.8-kg. dog was given 1.0 g. of acetophenetidin, there was a fall in blood pressure for 6 min., a rise to almost normal, and then a second drop. They estimated the lethal dose in this manner to be approximately 0.26 g. per kg. They observed no decrease in blood pressure in a curarized 15.8-kg. dog after the administration of 5.0 g. of the drug. They obtained a rise in blood pressure in dogs with the pneumogastric nerve cut, but no rise in blood pressure in a dog with the spinal cord and vagi cut. They concluded that moderate doses caused a rise in blood pressure by an effect on the heart and vasomotor system, that small doses increase the cardiac force and the pulse through cardiac stimulation, and that large doses decrease the pulse first through stimulating the cardio-inhibitory centers and later by a direct effect on the heart.

McGuigan (321) studied the effect of certain antipyretics on the toxicity of digitalis in dogs. A rise in blood pressure with a decrease in the fatal dose of digitalis was typical of all the antipyretics when they were given before the digitalis.

It is interesting to speculate on these early reports that acetophenetidin had a depressant effect on the heart. Speaking both of acetophenetidin and acetanilid, Sollmann (457) says they "may slow the heart indirectly by reducing the temperature; this has sometimes been misinterpreted as cardiac depression." Goodman and Gilman (160) says that "indeed, very large doses are required to affect adversely the heart or respiration" and that "only massive doses affect the heart and blood vessels directly." Others (449) observe that "however, their tendency to produce methemoglobin, with resulting cyanosis, led to the impression in early studies that the drugs had a deleterious effect on the circulation."

When one considers the problems of purification of acetophenetidin and the recent demonstration of toxic impurities (143), it is not surprising that the early studies sometimes revealed evidence of untoward effects that later were not confirmed by the use of pure material.

N-Acetyl-p-aminophenol. Hinsberg and Treupel (207) gave *N*-acetyl-*p*-aminophenol intravenously to a female rabbit weighing 1950 g. Two hours and 36 min. after beginning the experiment and after 4 g. of drug had been injected, the blood pressure rose from 97 to 114 mm. Hg and the pulse rate increased from 186 to 204 per min. After 3 hours, the blood pressure was 81 mm. and the pulse rate 186 per min. After 3 hours and 46 min., and after 6 g. of drug, the blood pressure was 45 mm. and the pulse rate 183 per min. After 4 hours the respiration stopped for 1 min., at which time the blood pressure was 28 mm. and the pulse 123 per min. Clark (74) perfused the coronary circulation of isolated rabbit hearts and found that doses of *N*-acetyl-*p*-aminophenol up to 25 mg. had little or no effect on the contractility or rate but did increase the coronary flow. Continuous intravenous infusion of up to 600 mg. per kg. in a dog produced only minor T-wave changes.

The available data suggest that acetophenetidin and *N*-acetyl-*p*-

aminophenol, even in relatively large doses, have no appreciable effect upon the heart or upon the blood pressure unless given intravenously at high concentrations.

Effects on Erythrocytes

Anemia

It was mentioned in the clinical literature as early as 1892 by Cleaves (75) that after continued administration of the drug, red corpuscles were destroyed and hemoglobin liberated with the resulting dark colored urine. West (512) remarked that after large doses of the drug, the red cells become shrunken and crenated with separation of the hematin. Davis (92) discussed the case of a woman who had taken acetophenetidin regularly for several months for the relief of headache. She had an anemia of undescribed degree which was, however, said to be less severe than the anemias described in cases of acetanilid poisoning. The possibility of an anemia of pregnancy was not excluded since she had not menstruated for 2 months. Krönig (256) described a 17-year-old printer's apprentice who had taken acetophenetidin in 1-g. doses, although apparently no more than four of these doses, in a 3-week period. After the fifth dose he became ill and hemolysis was observed. In a later paper Krönig (258) discusses the hemolysis in more detail. The red cells seemed to be dissolved with various degrees of solution visible. Some were changed in form with the hemoglobin remaining in the cell. In other instances the hemoglobin particles left the cell and dissolved in the serum or were taken up by the white blood cells in which they were deposited in the peripheral areas.

Poljakov (383) described the case of a 23-year-old man who on the day of admission had taken 60 g. of acetophenetidin within a period of 5 hours. Upon examination the erythrocyte count was 3.18 million per mm.^{3} Venesection was performed with a subsequent infusion of physiological saline solution. The second day after admission there was practically no change in the size of the erythrocytes but there were many normoblasts. By the third day there were 4 million erythrocytes and the hemoglobin index was 0.65, while on the fifth day there were still 4 million erythrocytes, but the hemoglobin was 58 per cent and the hemoglobin index was 0.72. Microscopic examination at this time revealed macrocytes and microcytes, and an irregular distribution of hemoglobin in the erythrocytes. Sometimes there were normoblasts and megaloblasts. On the sixth day the blood picture had changed showing many megalocytes, microcytes, and fragments of erythrocytes, as well as increased normoblasts and megaloblasts. On the seventh day the hemoglobin was 78 per cent and the erythrocytes 3.96 million. There were many fragments of erythrocytes and many normoblasts and megaloblasts. The normoblasts contained fragmented nuclei. On the eleventh day the erythrocyte count had dropped to 0.92 million per $mm.^3$ and on the twelfth day it was 0.91 million. On the thirteenth day there were signs of improvement in the blood with less poikilocytosis and anisocytosis. There were numerous normoblasts but very few megaloblasts. On the fourteenth day the hemoglobin was 14 per cent, and the erythrocytes 1.28 million per $mm.^3$ with a hemoglobin index of 0.93.

Storozhevoj (469) mentioned a 16-year-old girl who took 25 g. of the drug in the morning and that evening her erythrocyte count was 5.2 million with no morphological changes. On the sixth day she left the hospital, recovered and with an erythrocyte count of 3.7 million per $mm.^3$ In a review published in 1924, Lipschitz (283) mentioned that acetophenetidin probably produced less toxic effects on the blood than *N*-acetyl-*p*-aminophenol but he did not give any data. Reid (390) reported the case of a 28-year-old woman with a history of chronic acetophenetidin ingestion. Examination of the blood revealed a count of 2.74 million with a trace of poikilocytosis and moderate anisocytosis. There were no erythroblasts in a count of 200 cells.

In a 56-year-old woman who, for the past 38 years, had taken headache powders consisting of acetanilid, antipyrine, acetophenetidin, and caffeine, sometimes three or four a day, Clemmesen (76) observed that the erythrocyte count was 2.65 million, and the hemoglobin 47 per cent. In a 67-year-old woman who had taken acetophenetidin for about 30 years, Holst (213) observed a hemoglobin of 41 per cent and an erythrocyte count of 2.05 million per $mm.^3$

Hammarsten and Nordenfelt (178) discussed a case of chronic acetanilid and acetophenetidin toxicity in a 46-year-old woman. At the time of entrance to the clinic she had a hemoglobin of 95 per cent and an erythrocyte count of 4.6 million. She left the hospital after 1 month but returned at the end of 2 months after having taken the mixture of drugs again. She then had a hemoglobin of 90 per cent and the erythrocyte count was 4.0 million per $mm.^3$ Fourteen days after discontinuance of the drug the hemoglobin was 96 per cent and the erythrocyte count was 4.5 million. She had been taking a mixture of 0.1 g. acetanilid, 0.1 g. caffeine, 0.25 g. acetophenetidin, and 0.25 g. antipyrine. During attacks of migraine she took as much as 3 g. per day of the mixture and periodically took one powder every morning to get rid of headache.

Jasinski (229) describes the findings in a 20-year-old girl, schizophrenic, with suicidal tendencies, who took 20 to 30 tablets per day of an analgesic containing acetophenetidin. Upon admission to the hospital she had a hemoglobin of 63 per cent; in 5 weeks it rose to 82 per cent. The same author (230) describes 5 cases of toxic hemolytic anemia in women 22 to 54 years of age who had been taking 4 to 10 tablets of acetophenetidin daily for months or years. The anemia was hyperchromic and the per cent of reticulocytes was high. The serum iron was higher than normal and decreased as the patient recovered. After the administration of iron to these patients, the hemoglobin increased to normal and the lassitude and headaches disappeared. The author concluded that the toxic hemolytic anemia developed only because of an iron deficiency. Jasinski and Müller (231) described a case of a woman who had been taking, on her own initiative, a daily dose of 5 to 6 tablets, each containing 250 mg. acetophenetidin and 150 mg. isopropylantipyrine. When first examined her hemoglobin was 75 per cent and the erythrocytes 2.7 million. Reticulocytes were present in relatively high numbers. Eight days later the hemoglobin was 78 per cent and the erythrocytes 3.0 million. Reticulocytes still were 10 per cent. Upon sternal puncture the bone marrow was not abundant in cells. It contained reticule cells, 3 per cent, plasma cells, 1 per cent, neutrophiles, 8 percent, and myelocytes, 0 per cent. Thirty-five days after admission, the hemoglobin was 78 per cent, erythrocytes, 3.83 million, and reticulocytes, 4 per cent. Ninety-six days after the first examination the hemoglobin was 91 per cent, the erythrocytes, 4.68 million, and the reticulocytes, 8.8 per cent. The author concluded that these observations showed that chronic acetophenetidin administration did not necessarily cause a toxic hemolytic anemia. He believed that large doses of acetophenetidin in the male did not cause damage to the blood because there seldom was a primary iron deficiency in the male. The author mentioned another case of a housewife, 54 years old, who for approximately 10 years had taken 4 to 6 tablets daily of a mixture containing acetophenetidin. Her hemoglobin was 76 per cent, erythrocytes, 3.4 million, and reticulocytes, 38 per cent. Still another was a 41-year-old housewife who had a hemoglobin of 75 per cent with 3.1 million erythrocytes and reticulocytes, 5 per cent. The patient had been taking 2 to 4 tablets of the mixture daily for 3 months.

Fedotova and Khorsova (126) report that a woman with recurrent sharp headaches had taken for years as much as 40 powders, each containing 0.5 g. acetophenetidin and 0.5 g. aminopyrine. Her hemoglobin concentration was 20 per cent of normal and the reticulocyte count was 75 per cent. These values returned to normal after the drugs were discontinued.

Merlevede (325) reported the case of a woman, 39 years of age, who took 5 to 7 powders, each containing 0.35 g. acetophenetidin, 0.35 g. antipyrine, and 0.06 g. of caffeine, per day. She was treated by blood transfusions and the administration of ascorbic acid. Her hemoglobin rose from 65 per cent to 78 per cent, and the erythrocytes rose from 2.92 million to 3.84 million. She was all right for 4 years, at which time she returned after having used acetophenetidin again. She admitted having taken 14 powders on some days. She received iron, liver extract, and ascorbic acid and became well again. Another case was that of a woman 51 years of age who suffered from menopausal headaches. Her hemoglobin was 72 per cent, and the erythrocyte count 3.1 million. She had been taking 4 to 6 tablets per day of a mixture of 0.15 g. isopropyl antipyrine and 0.25 g. acetophenetidin. The patient recovered in a week after treatment with iron and ascorbic acid. The hemoglobin rose to 81 per cent, and the erythrocyte count to 4.6 million per $mm.^3$

In a recent study of 62 clinical cases of sulfhemoglobinemia, Brandenburg and Smith (44) found that out of the 7 patients who had been taking acetophenetidin none had a significant anemia. Schaub *et al.* (415), in discussing 27 cases of what they believed to be acetophenetidin intoxication, found that the blood was less saturated with oxygen and that the oxygen dissociation curve was shifted to the right, resulting in a decreased affinity for oxygen which in turn gave rise to cyanosis. They always observed a hypochromic anemia with macrocytosis as well as a reticulocytosis. They assumed that the drug exerted a direct toxic effect on the maturation of the erythrocytes in the bone marrow. The statement of Brown (51) that acetophenetidin causes depression of the bone marrow, or thrombocytopenia purpura, or both, is made without the presentation of any experimental data.

Horanyi (216) reported a serious anemia in two middle-aged women following the ingestion of large numbers of tablets containing acetophenetidin over a long period of time. Schwensen (427) described a 42-year-old woman who had taken 3 g. of acetophenetidin daily, and for 2 months even 4 to 5 g. daily. She also had been taking isonipecaine and barbiturates. Apparently because her hemoglobin was 66 per cent, she was diagnosed as having a hemolytic anemia due to acetophenetidin.

A few hours after taking 5 pills for a toothache, each containing 0.2 g. of acetophenetidin, 0.25 g. aminopyrine, 0.5 mgr. (*sic*) caffeine, and 0.05 g. quinine, a 22-year-old man suffered a severe hemolytic crisis, without cyanosis (414). The patient was not observed prior to ingesting the pills. Fifteen days later he still had a severe anemia which was accompanied by signs of rapid regeneration of blood corpuscles. In 35 days the anemia had regressed completely, and the patient was discharged from the hospital. Schweingruber (426) has studied 40 cases, including 32 women and 8 men who were reported to have taken mixtures containing acetophenetidin for a number of years. One-half of these patients had an anemia with hemoglobin concentrations of 27 to 78 per cent.

In a recent discussion of 35 cases of toxic hemolytic anemia after the administration of acetophenetidin, Wuhrmann and Jasinski (525) found that the bone marrow smears and peripheral blood counts were essentially normal or showed various degrees of anemia. Of the 35 cases 32 were women. They believe that an iron deficiency, more common in women, probably was a prerequisite for the appearance of the clinical manifestations and that the toxic hemolytic anemia which developed was a result of disturbances in the enzyme systems which detoxify and protect hemoglobin.

Selwyn (433) described the appearance of Heinz bodies in the erythrocytes of certain splenectomized patients. The Heinz bodies were believed to be particles of denatured methemoglobin, formed usually in mature erythrocytes, and occasionally in reticulocytes. In one patient, a 58-year-old woman who had had extensive surgery including splenectomy, and who had taken daily a few tablets each containing 0.25 g. aspirin, 0.25 g. acetophenetidin, and 0.008 g. of codeine phosphate, Heinz bodies were found in 20 per cent of the red cells. While she was in the hospital and no longer receiving the drug, the number fell to 3 per cent within a month and then gradually to 1.5 to 2.5 per cent in the next 2 months. She then began to take 2 tablets of the mixture three times a day, and the number of red cells with Heinz bodies rose to 25 per cent in 42 days and then later to 34 per cent. Another patient, a 45-year-old woman, who had had a partial gastrectomy and splenectomy 3 years before, had no Heinz bodies until she began taking tablets containing 0.3 g. acetophenetidin four times a day. After 16 days, 1.5 per cent of the erythrocytes had Heinz bodies. A 48-year-old man who had had a splenectomy had no Heinz bodies until he began taking 0.3-g. tablets of acetophenetidin four times a day for 14 days at which time 2 per cent of his erythrocytes had Heinz bodies. These persisted for 4 weeks while he continued to take acetophenetidin and then gradually disappeared after he stopped taking the drug. A 60-year-old man with probable splenic atrophy had no Heinz bodies in his erythrocytes but 3 weeks after he began taking 3 tablets a day, each containing 0.25 g. aspirin, 0.15 g. acetophenetidin, and 0.03 g. of caffeine, he had 1.4 per cent Heinz bodies.

A recent survey by Heck (193) of the adverse effects of drugs on blood lists acetophenetidin as one of many drugs reported to be associated with the production of blood dyscrasias, including hemolytic and aplastic anemias, but he gives no data.

One of the most significant contributions to the question of the acute hemolysis that is reported to occur occasionally after the administration of acetophenetidin and a number of other drugs is reported in a series of papers by Alving and co-workers. They (96) observed that the antimalarial drug, primaquine, produced a hemolytic anemia most frequently in American Negroes and even in an occasional Caucasian. They suggested that this is due to a defect in the older erythrocytes which also may cause sensitivity to acetophenetidin. They (97) designated as "sensitive" those subjects that exhibited significant hemolysis after the administration of 30 mg. primaquine daily. Erythrocytes from such individuals obtained after recovery from the effects of the drug were labeled with radiochromium and transferred into nonsensitive subjects who received the test drugs.

When acetophenetidin was given to such nonsensitive subjects, presumably at the rate of 0.3 g. every 4 hours for a total of 3.6 g., samples of labeled erythrocytes from 5 sensitive subjects were hemolyzed to the extent of 8 to 18 per cent, while samples from 3 subjects not sensitive to primaquine were not hemolyzed to a greater extent than 3 per cent. Subjects given acetanilid or primaquine hemolyzed the labeled cells 30 to 50 per cent.

They believe that such sensitive subjects may be detected on the basis of the *in vitro* formation in the erythrocytes of Heinz bodies by acetylphenylhydrazine (33). The defect, which occurs in about 10 per cent of American Negroes and rarely in Caucasians, is believed to be due to an abnormality affecting the activity of glucose-6-phosphate dehydrogenase (65).

N-Acetyl-p-aminophenol. In studies using erythrocytes from subjects sensitive to the hemolytic effects of primaquine (97), *N*-acetyl-*p*-aminophenol, presumably given in a dose of 0.3 g. every 4 hours for a total of 3.6 g., did not induce hemolysis to a significant extent.

It is difficult to assess the effect of acetophenetidin on the destruction of erythrocytes. Many of the older reports in the literature dealt with patients who were ill with various diseases and who had taken a number of different drugs. There are several reports of patients with various degrees of anemia after taking acetophenetidin, usually along with a number of other drugs, in relatively large doses over a period of several years. In more recent reports, most of the patients have been women, and the authors have suggested that many of them were suffering from an iron deficiency. The evidence suggests that, as Goodman and Gilman (160) write, "a hemolytic type of anemia can be produced, but the bone marrow is not depressed, and rapid and complete recovery occurs on cessation of medication."

Experimental Observations on Erythrocytes

Rats. Smith (446) gave adult albino rats daily doses of 720 mg. of acetophenetidin per kg., and at the end of 1 month withdrew blood 4 hours after administration of the last dose of the drug. He observed that the total hemoglobin was as high or perhaps slightly higher than it had been initially.

Wenzel *et al.* (510) have studied the effects of acetophenetidin on the sedimentation rate of the blood of rats. The rate was determined in male albino rats before administration of the drug and at weekly intervals thereafter for 3 weeks using the Cutler method. Blood was withdrawn by cardiac puncture. Groups of animals consumed a diet containing 0.1, 0.34, and 0.66 per cent of the drug, corresponding to daily doses of 60, 198, and 398 mg. per kg. Acetophenetidin had no consistent effect upon normal erythrocyte sedimentation.

Rabbits. Yustoff (526) in 1896 observed some anemia in rabbits and dogs given large doses of the drug for several days.

Dogs. In a dog given acetophenetidin, a decrease in the total oxygen content of the blood was observed (374,375).

Van Loon and Clark (495) administered acetophenetidin to 6 dogs in daily doses of 15 mg. per kg. for 43 to 150 days. Five of these animals were then continued on 30 mg. per kg. for 16 to 102 days, then 4 of the remaining animals continued on 60 mg. per kg. for 36 to 39 days, and finally 2 of the animals were continued on 120 mg. per kg. for 28 days. There was no change in fragility of the erythrocytes to hypotonic saline. The color and volume indices remained normal. The data suggested that doses of 60 and 120 mg. per kg. might produce a temporary decrease in hemoglobin and erythrocytes. During administration of the 60-mg. per kg. dose, there was a significant decrease in total hemoglobin, erythrocytes, and cell volume within the period of 15 days to 40 days but thereafter these values increased and were not significantly below the control values at the end of the experiment. With 120 mg. per kg., a significant decrease occurred during the period of 15 to 50 days followed by some increase in values. In both of these groups some increase in reticulocytes occurred after 21 to 28 days, which was significant in the 120-mg. per kg. group. Acetophenetidin was also administered in doses of 250 mg. per kg. for 15 days to 1 dog and for 100 days to 2 dogs, while doses of 200 mg. per kg. were given for 76 days to 2 dogs. The total hemoglobin, erythrocytes, and cell volume showed phasic decreases with a subsequent trend toward normal values. A decrease in erythrocyte counts was associated with reticulocytosis. During phases of anemia there was increase in volume index and a small increase in color index. It appears that in the dog probably 60 mg. per kg. of acetophenetidin is required to produce a sustained decrease in the erythrocytes in the peripheral blood and that the drug may produce a hemolytic anemia in sufficiently large or toxic doses. The data on the 250-mg. per kg. doses are illustrated in Figure 9.

Humans. Lester (274), using 15 male and 14 female subjects, gave 1 g. of acetophenetidin a day during the first 2 weeks, 2 g. a day during the third and fourth weeks in two 1-g. doses, and during the fifth and sixth week he gave 3 g. daily in equal doses at morning, noon, and evening. There was no decrease in total hemoglobin during the time the 1- and 2-g. doses were given, but there was a slight decrease during the 2 weeks when 3 g. were administered daily.

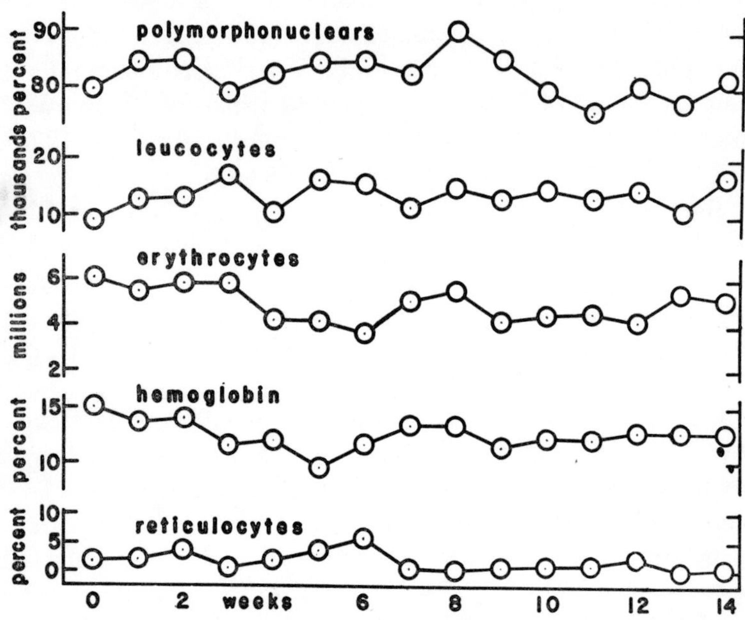

Figure 9. The effect of daily administration of acetophenetidin, 250 mg. per kg., on the blood morphology of dogs. (From Van Loon and Clark, ref. 495.)

Cyanosis

Cyanosis frequently is mentioned in the earlier literature as a clinical finding in patients after the administration of large doses of acetophenetidin. Occasionally this discoloration was due to altered blood pigments formed after the long-continued use of the drug. At other times it could be attributed to the low body temperature produced by very large doses of the drug in fever patients.

Early investigators observed that cyanosis depended a great deal on the dose. Hinsberg and Kast (206) noticed that after 2 to 3 doses of 0.5 g., there was no cyanosis. Lépine (271) stressed the absence of cyanosis after doses of 0.5 g., six to eight times a day. Éloy (117) reported that acetophenetidin administration frequently was accompanied by intense cyanosis and collapse. Dujardin-Beaumetz (104) said cyanosis was not observed, even with doses up to 3 g. Rohden (402) gave doses of 0.15 to 1.0 g. to adults and 0.1 to 0.2 g. to children and did not observe cyanosis, although Jaksch (237) did. Lindman (282), who gave a 34-year-old woman 1 g., followed by another gram the same morning, observed intense cyanosis of the fingernails, lips, and cheeks. By evening the patient felt better but was still slightly blue. Müller (345) observed that with doses of 8 g. per day there was cyanosis which ceased when the drug was discontinued. He did not believe that doses of 5 g. a day produced cyanosis. Rumpf (406) said that he never obtained cyanosis with doses of 1 g. Hollopeter (212) gave a 30-year-old woman acetophenetidin every 2 or 3 hours for a total of 12 doses of 0.5 g. each. Six hours later he observed marked cyanosis but the blueness did not last for more than 3 days. Popp (384) mentioned the case of a woman with migraine who received 1 g. of acetophenetidin and later took an additional gram and became cyanotic in the lips and cheeks.

Guleke (167) reported the case of a 48-year-old woman with fever who became quite cyanotic after taking 0.7 g. of acetophenetidin every 2 hours for a total of 7 g. Burkhalter (58) gave acetophenetidin for a total of 976 administrations to a total of 67 patients and observed 1 patient with typhus who became cyanotic after 0.75 g. of the drug. Tripold (488) gave doses of 0.2 to 0.3 g. of the drug and noticed one instance of marked cyanosis for 5 days after the drug was discontinued; he did not believe that there was any direct link between acetophenetidin administration and production of cyanosis. Collischonn (80) noticed that occasionally there was cyanosis after giving 1-g. doses four times a day. Rifat (397) observed cyanosis in one patient with typhoid fever who was receiving large doses of acetophenetidin. Demme (94) gave children, 2 to 4 years old, 0.1 to 0.2 g., those 5 to 11 years old, 0.2 to 0.5 g., and those 12 to 15 years old, 0.5 g. He observed a cyanotic coloration of the cheeks and mucous membranes in some of the patients. Cleaves believed that the drug produced profound cyanosis in many cases, but he did not cite the evidence. Betts (32) told of a patient who took 0.5 g. of acetophenetidin every 3 hours for 3 doses and whose face, after the third dose, became dark and swollen. West (512) stated that repeated or large doses of the drug cause cyanosis. Leech and Hunter (269) made a survey of physicians employing acetophenetidin and 3 of 220 reported that they had seen cyanosis at least once.

This occurred after doses ranging from 0.3 g. every 3 hours to 1.0 g. every 4 hours. An interesting case is mentioned by Cerna (69) in which a five-day-old child was given seven 0.15-g. acetophenetidin powders for diarrhea in the belief they were bismuth powders. The baby became fretful, weak, and purplish in color. The cyanosis continued for several days but the baby slowly recovered. The physician concluded that it undoubtedly was a case of pure acetophenetidin poisoning. Krönig (257) reported a fatal case of poisoning in which powders containing 0.1 g. of the drug had been taken for 3 weeks prior to the visit to the hospital. The patient was extraordinarily pale, but since he worked as a printer it was assumed that he had lead poisoning. When the pain did not stop he took more acetophenetidin. One morning the patient was extremely weak and cyanotic about the face and the lips. At this point acetophenetidin administration was stopped. The patient's body became more and more yellow in color and the lips, ears, hands, and feet were cyanotic. Eldridge (115) in reviewing the toxic symptoms resulting from administration of large doses of acetophenetidin, mentions cyanosis which was marked on the lips, face, and fingertips.

Greenleaf (163) described a 48-year-old woman with a headache who in 1 night took 5 powders, each containing 0.2 g. acetanilid, 0.2 g. acetophenetidin, and a little caffeine. She was observed to be weak, with extreme cyanosis especially around the fingers and lips. The cyanosis disappeared by the next day.

Löbl (285) tells of a 27-year-old law student who took 0.5-g. acetophenetidin powders during a severe attack of headache. He took one of these on an empty stomach and 30 min. later took another. About 1 hour after taking the last powder, a bluish color was at once strikingly apparent on the tip of the nose, the ears, fingertips, and membranes of the mouth. However, 3 hours after the first dose the cyanosis had decreased somewhat and another 3 hours later the cyanosis was evident only on the chin and fingernails. Meurice (327,328) describes cyanosis in a 48-year-old woman with facial neuralgia who took 11 g. of acetophenetidin in 20 hours. The cyanosis which was seen on the lips, cheeks, gums, and hands and feet, was particularly visible on the nails. By the next day the cyanosis had diminished, but even 4 days after taking the drug some evidence of it persisted. Russow (407) tells of a woman who had been perfectly healthy until 2 days before her death when she had noticed pain in her whole body after lightning had struck nearby. She was given 1 g. of acetophenetidin plus 0.2 g. of caffeine and sodium benzoate. In addition various other drugs were given such as camphor injections and 5-mg. doses of morphine. Two days after the pain developed, cyanosis of the face and extremities was observed, becoming extreme in the evening just before she died. It was not clear just how many doses of acetophenetidin she received.

Kebler *et al.* (238), in a survey of the harmful effects of acetophenetidin and certain other drugs, stated that of the 70 recorded cases in the medical literature, 34.3 per cent list cyanosis.

Storozhevoj (469) described a 16-year-old female patient who took 25 g. of acetophenetidin and developed cyanosis of the face and nails. By the following day the cyanosis of the face became quite noticeable especially in the ears. On the third day it diminished considerably and on the fourth day it had disappeared. Poljakov (383) described a 22-year-old man who, on the day of admission, had taken 60 g. of acetophenetidin during a period of 5 hours. Externally his skin and mucous membranes showed distinct signs of cyanosis with a pale-purple tinge. That evening his condition became worse, convulsions set in, and the cyanosis increased. The next day the cyanosis was still very marked, but it had almost disappeared on the eleventh day. Welsford (509) described a patient who took 5.8 g. of acetophenetidin within 1 hour. Two hours later he had marked cyanosis. The urgent symptoms passed within 3 hours but the cyanosis was still in evidence the next day. Hamill and Hine (176) reported the case of a 37-year-old woman who, contrary to instructions, took an unknown number of 0.3-g. tablets of acetophenetidin. She became violently ill and upon examination was a mauve color. The next day the cyanosis changed tint but did not disappear. By the following morning she was still blue in the lips, but felt better. Snapper (453) described cyanosis in a 63-year-old woman which increased in intensity for several days until her lips were dark blue. It was discovered that she had been given acetophenetidin for neuralgic pains in the arms and legs associated with a metastatic carcinoma. The drug was effective so the patient kept on taking it. In the last 4 months the daily dose had always been more than 1 g. After discontinuing the drug, cyanosis decreased and 3 months later was no longer noticeable. The drug was administered again and 3 days later there was intense cyanosis. He mentions a second case in a 57-year-old woman who had been given 0.5 g. of acetophenetidin four times a day for a year for neuralgic pains. In the clinic the cyanosis became better and had just about disappeared after 2 months. Ivens and van Vollenhoven (226) described a patient who was given acetophenetidin for more than 3 months and whose skin became discolored; the drug was discontinued. Reid (390) observed a 26-year-old woman admitted to the hospital for blueness of the fingers and finger tips. The blueness had appeared gradually about 6 weeks before and had been increasing until the patient's face became pale. There was a marked bluish tinge in the face and hands, and a very striking one in the lips, lobes of ears, fingertips, tongue, and mucous membranes. The patient had been taking acetophenetidin in large but unknown amounts for 5 months.

Harrop and Waterfield (188) observed cyanosis in a man who was believed to have been taking acetophenetidin, but this was not proved. Lundsteen *et al.* (293) reported the case of a 68-year-old man who, during the last 13 months, had taken four 1-g. tablets of acetophenetidin daily. Within the last 2 months his associates noticed a bluing of the face. At the time of hospitalization, he had a blue-black cyanosis which was marked on the cheeks, lips, tongue, and mucous membranes of the mouth, on the hands and on the nails. This disappeared after the use of the medicine was discontinued. Coxon and Crawford (1940) cited a patient with polyarthritis of 14 months' duration who had received daily doses of 0.2 to 1.2 g. acetophenetidin and who was strikingly cyanotic. There were no other ill effects observed and the authors state, "However, the patient has continued to take his phenacetin and is now as blue as ever, but apart from this and some disability resulting from his joint condition, he remains well and very contented."

Lesser (272) reported that acetophenetidin given over an extended period of time brings on symptoms of cyanosis and that the symptoms occur more frequently with acetanilid than with acetophenetidin.

A 20-year-old schizophrenic girl with suicidal tendencies took 20 to 30 tablets containing acetophenetidin per day causing her to be admitted to the hospital with extreme cyanosis of the mucous membranes (229). The patient recovered quickly without the use of medication, and the cyanosis decreased within a few days. Cerny (71) reported a 1-month-old child who was admitted to the hospital because of increasing cyanosis and collapse. When 3 weeks old she had suffered from cold and diarrhea, and the physician had ordered acetophenetidin. In 3 days the infant was given 3 suppositories containing a total of 1.8 g. of acetophenetidin. On the second day of the medication the mother noticed that the child became blue in color and was restless. In a second case, a 2-month-old girl was pale and cyanotic after having received 2 g. of acetophenetidin in suppositories. A third child became quite cyanotic after receiving a total of 3.8 g. acetophenetidin. A fourth case was that of an 11-month-old boy who had been given acetophenetidin in suppositories 2 days before admission to the hospital. A fifth case involved an 11-month-old girl who was given 12 suppositories of acetophenetidin in several days for a total of 3.6 g. There was a slight cyanosis of the face. Jasinski (230) reported 5 cases of cyanosis in women, 22 to 54 years of age, who had been taking 4 to 10 tablets of acetophenetidin a day for months or years. The cyanosis was in the lips and tongue and occasionally under the fingernails. There was no cyanosis of the cheeks, ears, or tip of nose. Jasinski and Müller (231) described 3 cases of chronic acetophenetidin ingestion with cyanosis of the lips and nails. Maier *et al.* (309) discussed 5 patients who had taken acetophenetidin for several months. All 5 had cyanosis. Schaub *et al.* (415,416), in describing acetophenetidin intoxication in 20 women and 4 men, said that all of them showed cyanosis with a gray or yellow-brown color which they ascribed to *p*-aminophenol. Wuhrmann and Jasinski (525) described 35 cases of hemolytic anemia in patients who had taken acetophenetidin among other forms of medications and observed that an ashen-gray cyanosis, especially of the mucous membranes and fingernail bed, did occur in these patients, even in the absence of any type of heart or lung disease.

Clemmesen (76) noticed cyanosis in a 56-year-old woman who had taken large doses of a mixture of acetanilid, antipyrine, acetophenetidin, and caffeine for 38 years. She often took 3 to 4 powders a day. Fisher (131) mentioned a 47-year-old man with tuberculosis who was admitted to the hospital in a markedly cyanotic condition. The patient admitted taking tablets, each containing 0.2 g. of acetophenetidin, in large numbers over a long period of time. He also took an effervescent preparation which apparently provided as much as 3.8 to 7.6 g. acetanilid daily. This habit was of 20 years' duration. At the time of admission it was estimated that he had been taking 8.4 g. acetanilid and 2.4 to 4.8 g. of acetophenetidin a day. Two months after withdrawal of the drugs his cyanosis had greatly diminished. Carter (66) observed marked cyanosis of the finger tips and lips in a woman who frequently took powders containing 0.5 g.

of acetophenetidin, 0.5 g. antipyrine, and 0.12 g. caffeine citrate for a total of 700 doses in less than a year. It was 2 months before the signs disappeared.

Archer and Discombe (14) mention the case of a woman, 48 years of age, who, after an operation for drainage of the sinuses, received 7.6 g. of acetophenetidin in 1 week and for the next 4 days received 3.0 g. of sulfanilamide daily. After only 7 g. of sulfanilamide had been given she became cyanotic. In another case, a 26-year-old woman in 15 days received 13 g. of acetophenetidin followed by 9 g. of sulfanilamide in 3 days. On the third day of sulfanilamide therapy there was a very slight cyanosis. It is obvious that the sulfanilamide probably was the major contributor to the cyanosis in these two cases.

Espersen (120) reports a case of a 30-year-old woman with marked cyanosis who had taken 1.5 g. acetophenetidin daily for 3 years. During the same interval she had taken many other drugs including bismuth, codeine, and phenobarbital. A patient of Schødt (422) with a headache had marked cyanosis and methemoglobin after having taken a mixture of 0.5 g. acetophenetidin and 0.05 g. caffeine. The case was complicated by pregnancy with intraperitoneal bleeding. Meulengracht and Lundsteen (326) discussed cyanosis in patients taking a mixture of 0.3 g. acetanilid, 0.3 g. antipyrine, 0.3 g. acetophenetidin, and 0.1 g. caffeine. The authors assumed that the cyanosis produced was most probably related to the intake of acetanilid. They mentioned that, even though acetophenetidin was related to acetanilid, similar findings had been observed only with ingestion of larger doses of acetophenetidin than these individuals had consumed.

Hammarsten and Nordenfelt (178) cite a 46-year-old woman who for the past 7 years regularly had taken powders which contained 0.1 g. acetanilid, 0.1 g. caffeine, 0.25 g. acetophenetidin, and 0.25 g. antipyrine. She took as much as 3 g. of the mixture a day and for the last 5 or 6 years had been cyanotic. After 1 month in the hospital the color diminished. Once dismissed, she began taking at least 2 headache powders a day, this time the powders were said to contain 0.1 g. caffeine, 0.3 g. acetophenetidin, and 0.3 g. antipyrine. Upon her second entry to the hospital her symptoms were the same as before with the lips, cheeks, and finger tips markedly cyanotic. Reissmann (391) reported the case of a 41-year-old woman who had once been a morphine addict and who subsequently took a mixture of codeine and acetophenetidin, 10 tablets a day at first, and 20 tablets a day for the last 4 years. She appeared pale with the lips a blue-gray color; her eyes were surrounded by light blue and she had cyanotic fingers and toes. The cyanosis was more pronounced on some days than on others. Lazarus (266) reports a housewife, aged 42, who was admitted to the hospital because of severe headache, weakness, and marked cyanosis. She had been taking tablets each containing 0.14 g. of acetophenetidin and 0.17 g. of aspirin over a period of 2 years. Sometimes she took as much as 4.2 g. acetophenetidin a day for headache, and in the 4 days before admission she had actually taken over 100 tablets. Merlevede (325) mentions the case of a 39-year-old woman with cyanotic lips, nails, and face who took 5 to 7 powders a day, each containing 0.35 g. acetophenetidin, 0.35 g. antipyrine, and 0.06 g. caffeine. She improved after treatment, and it was 4 years later when she returned with an even more intense cyanosis after having taken 12 to 14 powders a day. Horanyi (216) mentioned that cyanosis was present in a woman who had been taking large quantities of a mixture containing acetophenetidin over a long period of time. The methemoglobin content was only 1 g. per 100 ml. Schweingruber (426) listed a number of preparations containing acetophenetidin and related the cyanosis observed in patients to their total consumption of acetophenetidin. In 40 cases, cyanosis was present in 72 per cent.

DeSanctis *et al.* (98) observed a patient who was cyanotic despite the fact that she had no methemoglobin and only 0.8 g. of sulfhemoglobin per 100 ml. of blood. She had been taking numerous drugs, including one that gave a positive test for acetophenetidin. (In a later communication (107) it is stated that the indophenol reaction after hydrolysis was done, providing evidence that a drug of this class, not necessarily acetophenetidin, had been ingested.) Although she had had seven operations over the past 25 years and had been a surgical invalid for approximately 6 years, there was no record that her spleen had been removed.

It will be noted that reports of cyanosis after acetophenetidin administration were much more common in the early years when large doses were employed. More recent reports almost invariably associate cyanosis with the ingestion of large doses. As an instance of this there is the recent report (61) of a woman who took, with suicidal intent, 80 tablets of a mixture of drugs, containing a total of 4.0 g. acetophenetidin and 0.8 g. phenobarbital. Upon admission to the hospital, 5 hours later, she was described as being very sleepy and intensely cyanotic although only 15 per cent of her hemoglobin was methemoglobin. By the next day the cyanosis had disappeared. Cyanosis is not observed after the ingestion of moderate doses.

Experimental Observations of Cyanosis

In a very early study Hinsberg and Kast (206) showed that when a dog received a dose of 3 to 5 g. of acetophenetidin there was a definite cyanosis of the mucous membranes of the mouth. Mahnert (307) reported that when a rabbit weighing 650 g. was fed 2.5 g. acetophenetidin the mucous membranes and skin became cyanotic. Cyanosis usually developed when the drug was administered by various routes to guinea pigs, rabbits, white mice, and dogs (267). Hamill and Hine (176) observed that when a 1.6-kg. albino rabbit was given 0.35 g. of acetophenetidin intraperitoneally there was no cyanosis of the ears or eyes visible by daylight. Rosen (403) stated that 1 g. killed a live healthy rabbit in 76 min. and that cyanosis was a prominent symptom. The nasal mucous membrane of a 1.92-kg. cat given 0.4 g. of drug per kg. was slightly blue after 40 min. and there was strong cyanosis after 3 hours, but by the next day the mucous membranes were pink (203). Löbl (285) found that doses of 2 to 5 g. in the dog can cause serious symptoms of poisoning including cyanosis. There was light cyanosis after 90 to 120 min. in a dog given 0.5 to 1.0 g. per kg. of the drug (207).

Brownlee (53) gave male rats weighing 120 to 150 g. daily doses of acetophenetidin equivalent to 25 per cent of the LD_{50}, which a previous study (54) had shown to be 1250 mg. per kg. A cyanosis developed but it passed off in the course of 6 to 8 hours. Hambourger (175) gave acetophenetidin to rats in doses of 4 to 6 g. per kg. by stomach tube and reported that death seemed to be due to some sort of blood dyscrasia which was associated with cyanosis.

It is well to remember that, both in the clinical cases and experimental animals, cyanosis refers merely to a blue appearance. In itself it is not an adequate sign of drug intoxication and, indeed, may be unrelated to its principal pharmacological and toxicological actions.

Occurrence of Methemoglobin in Patients

Müller (346) observed that, in one case of pulmonary tuberculosis and in another of facial erysipelas, the administration of 6 to 8 g. of acetophenetidin daily was associated with methemoglobinemia, which was not however accompanied by collapse and disappeared when the drug was discontinued. He suggested that cyanosis and methemoglobinemia probably could have been avoided by giving doses no larger than 5 g. a day, which is still far in excess of the dose recommended at the present time. Müller (345) reports that doses of 8 g. a day were not without danger and might be associated with methemoglobinemia. Tripold (488) listed one patient in whom there were very disagreeable side-effects, and a blood examination revealed methemoglobin. However this was observed at a time when the drug had not been given for 5 days, so he concluded that there was no direct link between the acetophenetidin and its occurrence.

Brunton (56), in his lectures on the action of medicines, mentioned that all drugs such as acetophenetidin have the property of forming methemoglobin. Löbl (285) mentioned a law student, aged 27 years, who had methemoglobinemia after taking 1 powder of acetophenetidin on an empty stomach. He did not mention actually finding methemoglobin in this patient but said that in animal studies it is possible to detect its accumulation. Meurice (327,328) cited the case of a 48-year-old woman who took 11 g. of acetophenetidin in about 20 hours. He mentioned that, even on the next day, the complexion was darker due to methemoglobinemia. Russow (407) wrote of a woman who was normal and healthy until she suddenly noticed pain in her whole body after lightning struck nearby. She was treated for the pain with two doses in one day, each containing 1 g. acetophenetidin and 0.2 g. caffeine sodium benzoate. A spectroscopic analysis of the filtered and freshly voided urine showed the dark methemoglobin band between the orange and yellow ones.

The blood of a student who during a 5 hour period took 60 g. of acetophenetidin was almost a black color when examined spectroscopically the second day and contained methemoglobin (383). Stadie (465), enumerating those agents which changed hemoglobin to methemoglobin, included acetophenetidin among them, but he gave no experimental data on this drug. Fisher (131) described a patient, a man aged 47, who took 2.4 to 4.8 g. of acetophenetidin and 3.8 to 7.6 g. of acetanilid daily over a long period of time. Spectroscopic examination of the blood revealed methemoglobin in large amounts. Lundsteen *et al.* (294) described a case of chronic acetophenetidin intoxication in a 62-year-old male, who during the last year, took four 1-g. tablets of acetophenetidin daily. At the time of hospitalization he had cyanosis, but spectroscopic examination of the blood failed to reveal methemoglobin. Reissmann (391) reported a case of a 41-year-old woman who had once been a morphine addict but who had subsequently taken a mixture of codeine and acetophenetidin regularly for the last 7 years. In the first 3 years she took 10 such tablets per day, and in the last 4 years twice as many. There was some methemoglobin present but the degree of methemoglobinemia seemed to be unrelated to the dose of acetophenetidin, provided that there was more than a minimal amount. Finch (130) reviewed the literature on the production of methemoglobinemia due to drugs, including acetophenetidin, but he did not give any original data. Cerny (71) mentioned 5 cases of children who had been given acetophenetidin in various doses. He observed cyanosis in all of them and he concluded that they had methemoglobinemia. In a recent study of 62 clinical cases of sulfhemoglobinemia reported by Brandenburg and Smith (44), they found that there was methemoglobinemia in 49 cases, but in only 1 of these was there any evidence that the patient had taken acetophenetidin. In the 24 cases reported by Schaub *et al.* (415,416), most of whom had been taking excessive doses of acetophenetidin, all patients showed cyanosis and evidence of sulfhemoglobinemia, but methemoglobin was present in only 1.

Contaminated materials. There is an interesting report in 1950 by Hald (171) of the use of a batch of acetophenetidin contaminated with 18 per cent of *p*-chloracetanilid. All of the patients exhibited methemoglobinemia. Schmith and Madsen (421) observed 4.2 per cent methemoglobin in a woman 4 hours after she had taken 8 tablets of the contaminated acetophenetidin in 13 hours.

Gad *et al.* (143) described other cases of methemoglobinemia after taking the contaminated acetophenetidin. He also gave subjects 10 mg. of *p*-chloracetanilid and found 1 to 2 per cent methemoglobin in the blood. The finding that as little as 10 mg. of this contaminant could produce a significant methemoglobinemia suggests that it may have been a rather common impurity in the early years and probably was responsible for the more frequent mention of methemoglobin formation in the early literature.

Mixtures containing acetophenetidin. Jasinski and Müller (231) described a patient who habitually took a number of tablets containing 0.25 g. acetophenetidin and 0.15 g. isopropyl antipyrine. This woman had various blood changes but no pigments were found by spectroscopic examination of the plasma. In hemolyzed blood there was a pathological pigment with an absorption band between 608 and 624 mμ which could be observed at a dilution up to 1:30. This absorption band could not be extinguished with sodium sulfite. The pigment was distinguishable from methemoglobin since its absorption band lies at 630 mμ and is wider. Merlevede (325) cites a 39-year-old woman who had taken powders containing 0.35 g. acetophenetidin, 0.35 g. antipyrine, and 0.06 g. caffeine for the past 13 years for headache. She usually took 1 to 2 powders a day but recently took 5 to 7. The blood spectrum showed an absorption band at 630 mμ which diminished after the addition of ascorbic acid and sodium hydrosulfite; these reagents also changed the absorption at 620 mμ. It was therefore suggested that sulfhemoglobin was present along with the methemoglobin. He mentioned also a 51-year-old woman who took 4 to 6 tablets a day, each containing 0.15 g. isopropyl antipyrine and 0.25 g. acetophenetidin. The blood showed light absorption at 625 mμ, which completely disappeared after the addition of ascorbic acid and sodium hydrosulfite. Schaub *et al.* (416) observed that the blood of 20 women and 4 men, who were said to have taken large doses of acetophenetidin for a long time, contained inactive hemoglobin, 0.3 to 1.6 g. per cent, in all cases. Horanyi (216) observed that there were 1.1 g. per cent and 1.4 g. per cent methemoglobin, respectively, in 2 patients who had been taking a mixture containing acetophenetidin and that cyanosis was observed in 1 of them. A recent report of a woman who took 4.0 g. of acetophenetidin plus 0.8 g. phenobarbital and some other drugs revealed only 15 per cent methomoglobin (61).

Methemoglobin formation has been associated with the ingestion of large doses of acetophenetidin or smaller doses of the contaminated drug. It is rare in individuals taking moderate doses, even for a long period of time.

It will be noted that, in many of the early clinical reports, there were inadequate demonstrations of the presence of methemoglobin and it was not well differentiated from other pigments.

Experimental Production of Methemoglobin

Rats. Smith (445) gave daily doses of 720 mg. acetophenetidin per kg. to rats and observed that it produced almost equal quantities of methemoglobin and sulfhemoglobin. Smith (446) found that this dose of acetophenetidin suspended in 2 per cent acacia solution and given by stomach tube to 8 albino rats for 1 month resulted in 1.6 g. methemoglobin per 100 ml.; the control rats had 0.3 mg. per 100 ml. A molecular equivalent dose of *p*-aminophenol gave rise to only 0.08 g. of methemoglobin per 100 ml.

In the studies on acetophenetidin contaminated with 18 per cent *p*-chloroacetanilid, Gad *et al.* (143) showed that 30 mg. of the contaminant per rat produced at least 5 per cent methemoglobin in almost all of the animals. In 15 rats the average methemoglobin was about 25 per cent of the total blood pigment.

Rabbits. Mahnert (307) observed that large doses of acetophenetidin produced methemoglobin in rabbits. Hamill and Hine (176) gave a 1600-g. albino rabbit 0.35 g. of acetophenetidin intraperitoneally, and this animal showed no spectroscopic evidence of methemoglobin in blood samples taken at intervals after the injection.

Dogs. Hinsberg and Kast (206) gave dogs weighing 5 to 6 kg., 3 to 5 g. of acetophenetidin a day for several days and observed a definite cyanosis with methemoglobin present irregularly in the blood. Hinsberg and Treupel (207) gave dogs 0.5 to 1.0 g. per kg. and noticed that after 2.5 hours there were methemoglobin bands in the blood. Dennig (95) observed that acetophenetidin *in vitro* did not produce methemoglobin within a 36 hour period. He gave a dog 408 mg. of acetophenetidin per kg. and noticed that the maximum methemoglobin formation of 42 per cent occurred 5 hours later and that the level returned to normal after 25 hours. In another experiment in which the dog vomited most of a 1.0 g. per kg. dose, the maximal methemoglobin of 36 per cent was seen at 5.5 hours. He suggested that recovery was possible after 60 per cent methemoglobin formation. Overlach (362) gave a dog 1.0 g. of acetophenetidin per kg. and observed the typical spectrum of methemoglobin. Methemoglobin was noticeable in the blood 3 hours after Heubner (203) gave a dog 2.5 millimoles of acetophenetidin per kg. Piccinini (376) was unable to detect methemoglobin after the administration of 429 mg. per kg. to dogs.

Van Loon and Clark (495) gave acetophenetidin to 6 dogs in a dose of 15 mg. per kg. for from 43 to 150 days. Five of these animals were continued on 30 mg. per kg. for 16 to 102 days, and then 4 of them on 60 mg. per kg. for 39 to 46 days. Finally 2 of the animals received 120 mg. per kg. for 28 days. The minimal dose producing temporary methemoglobinemia in the dog was 30 mg. per kg. Its duration was related to the quantity of drug administered. No more than traces were present 20 hours after the largest dose. There was no accumulation of methemoglobin.

In the dog, the amount of methemoglobin formation showed a correlation with the plasma *p*-phenetidin levels found after the administration of large doses of either acetophenetidin or *p*-phenetidin (48). With doses of acetophenetidin of 75 mg. per kg., the maximum methemoglobin was 32 per cent in one animal and 33 per cent in another. With *p*-phenetidin in a dose of 12 mg. per kg., the maximum methemoglobin was 45 per cent in one and 47 per cent in another. The data are presented in Table 4.

TABLE 4

Correlation of *p*-Phenetidin and Methemoglobin Levels in the Blood after Administration of *p*-Phenetidin and Acetophenetidin to Dogs (From Brodie and Axelrod, ref. 48)

Dog	Drug	Dose, mg./kg.	*p*-Phenetidin, maximum plasma levels, mg./liter	Methemoglobin, maximum %
1	Acetophenetidin	75	4.3	32
2	Acetophenetidin	75	5.2	33
3	*p*-Phenetidin	12	5.0	45
4	*p*-Phenetidin	12	6.6	47

Cats. Heubner (203) gave a 1.9-kg. cat, 0.4 g. of acetophenetidin, and after 1.5 hours the blood from the ear was very dark and showed methemoglobin. Lewis (277) gave orally to 4 cats, 0.2 millimoles of acetophenetidin per kg. and found 3 per cent methemoglobin after 3 hours in one animal, but none in the other 3. Renault *et al.* (393) found that a dose of 0.3 millimole per kg. converted 33.5 per cent of the hemoglobin to methemoglobin.

Various species. Lester (273) studied the maximum amounts of methemoglobin produced by single doses of acetophenetidin in rats, cats, rabbits, dogs, monkeys, and man. Food was withheld for 16 hours before and 5 hours after the drug was given to the animals by stomach tube as a 2 per cent acacia suspension. Blood was withdrawn at 1 hour intervals after administration, and total hemoglobin, methemoglobin, and sulfhemoglobin were determined. The minimal or threshold dose of acetophenetidin required to produce methemoglobin in man was about 0.084 millimoles per kg. corresponding to 1 g. in an average-sized man. He concluded that in the rabbit and monkey there was virtually no methemoglobin formation and that man was slightly more than $^1/_2$ as sensitive as the cat, the dog $^1/_2$ as sensitive as man, and the rat $^1/_6$ as sensitive as the dog. Some of the data are presented in Figure 10.

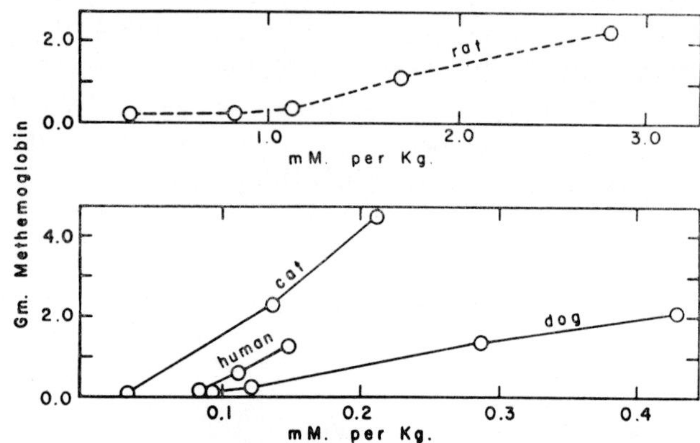

Figure 10. Species differences at maximum formation of methemoglobin for various doses of acetophenetidin. (From Lester, ref. 273.)

Human. Brodie and Axelrod (48) gave subjects acetophenetidin and determined the methemoglobin at intervals over an 8 hour period. The methemoglobin formation was maximal 3 hours after administration. The results are presented in Table 5.

TABLE 5

Plasma Acetophenetidin and Per Cent Methemoglobin Following Oral Administration of Acetophenetidin to Man. (From Brodie and Axelrod, ref. 48)

Time, hr.	Subject A (1.2 g.) Acetophenetidin, mg./l.	Subject A (1.2 g.) Methemoglobin, %	Subject B (2.0 g.) Acetophenetidin, mg./l.	Subject B (2.0 g.) Methemoglobin, %	Subject C (2.0 g.) Acetophenetidin, mg./l.	Subject C (2.0 g.) Methemoglobin, %
1	0.7	0.3	4.9	1.2	1.4	0.6
2	2.2	0.8	4.0	1.2	0.8	0.6
3	0.7	1.3	2.2	2.4	0.3	3.3
5	0.2	1.0	1.1	1.9	0.05	1.4
8	0.1	1.3	0.2	1.7	0.0	1.4

N-Acetyl-p-aminophenol. The question of methemoglobin formation after large doses of *N*-acetyl-*p*-aminophenol was investigated by the oral administration of this compound to albino rats in doses of 1.0, 2.0, and 4.0 g. per kg. (162). Frequent determinations of methemoglobin over a period of 8 hours showed that none was formed in any of the animals. Although white rats are not sensitive to methemoglobin forming compounds, they did show approximately 13 per cent methemoglobin after the oral administration of 200 mg. of acetanilid per kg. Clark (74) found no significant amounts of methemoglobin in rats after 3200 to 3600 mg. of *N*-acetyl-*p*-aminophenol per kg. A dose of 100 mg. *N*-acetyl-*p*-aminophenol per kg. in a dog produced 3.2 g. methemoglobin per 100 ml. blood after 2.75 hours. In another dog a dose of 200 mg. per kg. produced 4.7 g. methemoglobin per 100 ml. after 4.75 hours. This difference between the effect in dogs and in rats is probably a species difference, since it is known that dogs are rather sensitive to the effects of methemoglobin forming compounds.

Renault *et al.* (393) found that a dose of 0.3 millimole per kg. produced only 1.7 per cent methemoglobin in cats and that as much as 2.0 millimole per kg. was necessary to convert 50 per cent of the hemoglobin to methemoglobin. This was more than twice the dose of acetophenetidin required to produce the same effect.

Free *et al.* (138) studied the effect of *N*-acetyl-*p*-aminophenol upon the production of methemoglobin in dogs. Doses of 100 mg. per kg. produced only barely detectable amounts. Doses of 150 mg. per kg. caused the formation of about 10 per cent methemoglobin, and oral or intravenous doses of 250 mg. per kg. produced about 30 per cent after 2 to 4 hours. This had largely disappeared after 13 hours. When a dog was given 1000 mg. per kg. orally, the methemoglobin was 11.9 g. per cent or 77 per cent of the total blood pigment at the end of 7 hours and the animal died 3 hours later.

Greenberg and Lester (162) gave each of 2 normal human subjects in the post-absorptive state 1.09 g. of *N*-acetyl-*p*-aminophenol orally. No methemoglobin was found in blood samples taken 1, 2, and 6 hours afterwards. Boréus and Sandberg (37,39) gave 3 g. of *N*-acetyl-*p*-aminophenol or of acetophenetidin to medical students and found that the maximal methemoglobin 3 hours later was 0.13 g. per 100 ml. after the former compound, and 0.4 g. per 100 ml. after acetophenetidin. The results are illustrated in Figure 11.

Occurrence of Sulfhemoglobin in Patients

Sulfhemoglobin is a poorly defined blood pigment distinguished from methemoglobin by a different absorption spectrum and greater

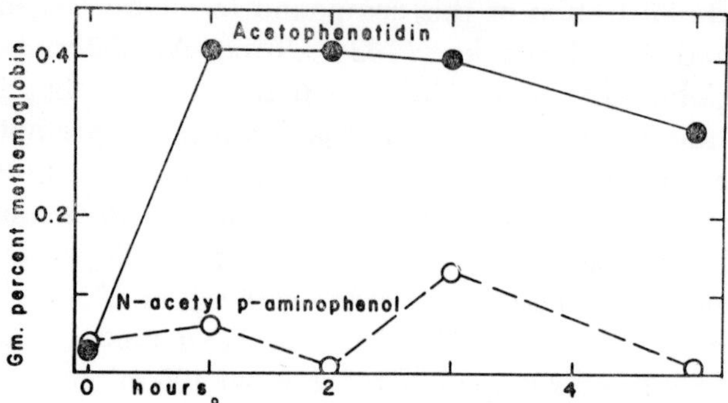

Figure 11. Mean values of methemoglobin in four subjects after the administration of 3 g. acetophenetidin or *N*-acetyl-*p*-aminophenol. (From Boréus and Sandberg, ref. 37.)

chemical inertness. Gibson (152) mentions that sulfhemoglobin is formed in the presence of hydrogen sulfide produced by intestinal bacteria and in the presence of acetophenetidin and other drugs, but he gives no experimental data. He believes that the sulfhemoglobin iron is present in the ferrous form but that it does not combine reversibly with oxygen. Sulfhemoglobin does not occur in normal blood, and apparently there is no mechanism for converting it to hemoglobin as there is in the case of methemoglobin.

Snapper (452) was one of the first to study the incidence of sulfhemoglobin after the administration of drugs. Some of the patients he observed had received acetophenetidin. Ivens and van Vollenhoven (226) discussed two kinds of cyanosis, one due to methemoglobin and one to sulfhemoglobin. They presented the history of a patient who had complained of mysterious stomach pains and who was given acetophenetidin over a period of 3 months. Since he developed skin discoloration, the drug was discontinued, but 4 months later the skin and mucous membranes still were a blue-gray color. This they believed was due to sulfhemoglobinemia because the blood showed the red band and characteristic reactions as described by van den Bergh. They believed that in this patient acetophenetidin had produced sulfhemoglobinemia. In various patients with liver dysfunction they were able to produce sulfhemoglobinemia with the administration of sulfur alone, but they obtained it much more readily if acetophenetidin also was given. They concluded that acetophenetidin enhanced the production of sulfhemoglobin by sulfur in the intestinal contents but that its presence was not necessarily required. Other reducing substances would do likewise, particularly in patients with liver dysfunction. Snapper (453) said that the hemoglobin was sensitized by acetophenetidin so that sulfhemoglobin was easily produced in the intestinal wall. The blood from the intestine then circulated to the liver where the sulfhemoglobin was broken down. The decomposition took place readily in the normal liver but only with difficulty in the diseased liver so that in this case some of the sulfhemoglobin was returned unchanged into the general circulation. He described a case of a 63-year-old woman admitted to the hospital with a diagnosis of cancer with metastases. Cyanosis was first observed after she had been in the clinic for 9 months. It increased in intensity and in several days the lips were dark-blue. Spectroscopic analysis of the blood revealed a strong spectral band at 615 mμ, which remained after the addition of ammonium sulfide, indicating that it was due to sulfhemoglobin. It was discovered meanwhile that the patient had been given acetophenetidin for neuralgic pains in the arms and legs. This treatment was so successful that the patient kept on taking the drug, the dose varying from 0.5 to 1.5 g. per day. In the last 4 months the daily dose had always been more than 1 g. When it was discovered that the patient had sulfhemoglobinemia she was put on a milk diet but acetophenetidin administration was continued. The cyanosis was no better after 2 weeks, and the spectroscopic appearance of the blood was unchanged. When acetophenetidin administration was stopped both the cyanosis and the sulfhemoglobin content of the blood decreased until after 1 month the sulfhemoglobin band was much less intense. A second case was that of a 50-year-old woman, also cyanotic. A spectroscopic analysis showed a red band which remained after the addition of ammonium sulfide. The patient had tabes and had taken 0.5 g. of acetophenetidin four times a day for 1 year for neuralgic pain. In the clinic acetophenetidin was not administered, and the cyanosis became weaker until after 4 months none could be detected. In 6 patients with normal intestinal function the administration of 0.5 g. acetophenetidin three times a day for 10 days produced a definite sulfhemoglobinemia. Methemoglobinemia was not observed in these cases, not even in experiments which lasted several weeks. When acetophenetidin and sulfur were administered at the same time, sulfhemoglobinemia was produced readily in many patients but not in all. It was produced most readily in patients who had liver dysfunction in whom 1.5 g. of acetophenetidin per day, with or without 2 g. of precipitated sulfur, produced the strong sulhemoglobin band in 2 or 3 weeks. Snapper believed that acetophenetidin produced an increased sensitivity of the hemoglobin so that, with even a small increase in the hydrogen sulfide content of the intestine, the sensitized pigment was converted to sulfhemoglobin. Harrop and Waterfield (188) described a man whom they considered an unreliable witness, who said he had taken only aspirin for 4 years. They suggested that he also might have taken acetophenetidin without knowing it. He suffered from habitual extreme headaches and developed sulfhemoglobinemia unaccompanied by methemoglobinemia. They also confirmed Snapper's observation in dogs that small doses of acetophenetidin and sulfur given simultaneously resulted in sulfhemoglobin formation in a few days. The sulfhemoglobin, once produced, persisted for days without any appreciable diminution. Weeks elapsed before it all had disappeared from the blood. Healy (192) reviewed some of the literature on sulfhemoglobinemia and concluded that acetophenetidin in large doses in the presence of hydrogen sulfide gave rise to sulfhemoglobin. He cited two cases involving acetanilid but none involving acetophenetidin.

Lundsteen *et al.* (294) described sulfhemoglobin formation in chronic acetophenetidin poisoning in a 62-year-old man who had taken acetophenetidin tablets daily during the preceding 13 months. A patient with arthritis of 14 months' duration who received daily doses of 0.2 to 1.2 g. acetophenetidin was strikingly cyanotic, and spectroscopic examination revealed the characteristic band of sulfhemoglobin in the blood 6 months after admittance at which time, however, he was still taking acetophenetidin (86). In reviewing the action of various drugs which produced altered blood pigments, Hanzlik (180) pointed out that if cyanosis persisted, the darkening of the blood had to be due to some pigment other than methemoglobin, such as sulfhemoglobin or coal-tar oxidation products. Von Oettingen (499) reviewed the evidence that acetophenetidin favored sulfhemoglobin formation, especially in persons suffering from injury to the liver. In addition he described its occurrence in an adult 71-kg. male given acetophenetidin in 3 doses of 1 g. each at intervals of approximately 4 hours.

A 42-year-old housewife, admitted to the hospital because of weakness and cyanosis for a period of 2 years, had taken sometimes as many as 30 tablets a day each containing 0.15 g. of acetophenetidin and 0.25 g. aspirin (266). In the 4 days before admission she ingested over 100 tablets. Upon admission the blood showed absorption in the red portion of the spectrum at 612 to 620 mμ. This was detectable in a 1:100 dilution of blood even 2 days after admission and was presumed to be due to sulfhemoglobin. The blood of a male patient, 57 years of age, who had taken 16 g. of acetophenetidin in 2 weeks contained sulfhemoglobin which was easily detected in a 1:65 dilution. Finch (130) said that acetophenetidin was among those drugs causing sulfhemoglobinemia, but he presented no data. Kiese (240) mentions that acetophenetidin, among other drugs, gave rise to the production of verdiglobin which may be identical with sulfhemoglobin. He did not give any experimental data on the production of this pigment by acetophenetidin.

Jasinski and Müller (231) cited the case of a woman who had been taking tablets containing acetophenetidin. Examination of the blood revealed no pigments in the plasma but they were present in the hemolyzed blood. A 54-year-old housewife, who for approximately 10 years had taken 4 to 6 tablets of an acetophenetidin mixture daily, had a pigment absorbing at 620 mμ in a 1:10 dilution of hemolyzed blood. A similar pigment was present in the blood of a 47-year-old housewife who had been taking 2 to 4 tablets of an acetophenetidin mixture daily for a long time. Maier *et al.* (309) described 5 patients in whom a blood absorption band between 620 and 640 mμ was recorded which could not be removed with sodium hydrosulfide and which, they therefore decided, was due to sulfhemoglobin. These patients had been taking acetophenetidin. When the oxygen tension of the blood was plotted against the oxygen pressure, the values for acetophenetidin patients were on the right of the curve, whereas the values for patients receiving nitrite were on the normal curve. They believed that there was a difference between the dyscrasias caused by acetophenetidin and by nitrite, and that these drugs do not produce the same sort of methemoglobinemia.

Brandenburg and Smith (44) reported evidence of sulfhemoglobin in 82 cases but only 62 were actually studied. Of these 7 were attributed to mixtures containing acetophenetidin.

Merlevede (325) described the findings in a 39-year-old woman who had been taking daily 5 to 7 powders containing 0.35 g. acetophenetidin combined with antipyrine and caffeine. The absorption band at 630 mμ disappeared partially after addition of ascorbic acid and sodium hydrosulfide but another band appeared at 620 mμ. He suggested that there was sulfhemoglobin along with methemoglobin. In a 51-year-old woman who had taken 4 to 6 tablets of a mixture containing 0.25 g. of acetophenetidin and 0.15 g. of isopropylantipyrine, the blood showed absorption at 625 mμ which disappeared completely after addition of ascorbic acid and sodium hydrosulfide with a new band appearing at 618 mμ. The author surmised that this was due to sulfhemoglobin. In the 24 cases reported as acetophenetidin intoxication by Schaub *et al.* (415), they observed that there was an absorption band at 619 mμ in the blood which was not reduced with potassium cyanide. They considered it to be sulfhemoglobin or verdiglobin. Wuhrmann and Jasinski (525) in their cases of toxic hemolytic anemia after acetophenetidin observed also that those patients with sulfhemoglobinemia did not show rapid reversion of the pigment to hemoglobin as did patients with methemoglobinemia.

DeSanctis *et al.* (98) described a 43-year-old woman, a former shoe-factory employee, who had bouts of nausea, vomiting, and turning blue for a period of 4 days and had 4 similar episodes during the past 6 years. For the last 3 years she also had intermittent diarrhea. There was some evidence that she had chronic ulcerative colitis (444). She had had numerous and extensive surgical operations over the past 25 years and had been a surgical invalid for the past 6 years. Her total hemoglobin was 10.4 g. per 100 ml., and it was calculated that approximately 0.8 g. of this was sulfhemoglobin. No methemoglobin was detected. She had been taking numerous drugs including one that was said to have given a positive test for acetophenetidin in the urine. In a later communication, one of the authors (107) stated that they tested the urine by the well-known indophenol reaction after hydrolysis, thus providing presumptive proof of ingestion of one of this class of compounds.

Experimental Studies of Sulfhemoglobin

Rats. Smith (445) gave 720 mg. of acetophenetidin per kg. daily to rats for 1 month and found that it produced detectable quantities of sulfhemoglobin. At the end of 1 month (446) there was 0.5 g. of sulfhemoglobin per 100 ml. of blood in the treated animals. Recently Silver *et al.* (437) studied the rate of disappearance of sulfhemoglobin after its experimental production. Rabbits were given daily doses of 0.75 g. acetophenetidin plus an equal amount of precipitated sulfur for 1 to 4 weeks. The sulfhemoglobin formed disappeared at the rate of 8 per cent a week.

Dogs. Snapper (452) gave acetophenetidin to dogs and observed the production of sulfhemoglobin. Van Loon and Clark (495) gave acetophenetidin to dogs in doses of 15 mg. per kg. and then increased the dose progressively to 30 and finally to 120 mg. per kg. There was no accumulation of sulfhemoglobin in these animals. Doses of 13 to 28 mg. acetophenetidin per kg. plus 14 to 22 mg. precipitated sulfur per kg. plus, in some cases, potassium sulfide, changed as much as 20 per cent of the hemoglobin of dogs to sulfhemoglobin. Formation of sulfhemoglobin was less rapid after acetophenetidin administration than after giving *p*-aminopropiophenone or trinitrotoluene. Erythrocytes of these dogs, labeled with Fe^{55} and transfused into normal dogs, did not disappear more rapidly than erythrocytes containing no sulfhemoglobin.

Kallner (235) did some interesting experiments which caused him to question the usual findings of methemoglobin and sulfhemoglobin after large doses of acetophenetidin. He added the drug to untreated blood and found that there was no change in absorption spectra if the blood had been aerated. However, if the blood had been taken under oil there was increased absorption at 623, 617, and 610 mμ. He believed this was due to the presence of a labile compound with carbhemoglobin which, of course, required carbon dioxide for its formation. This compound did not affect the oxygen carrying capacity of the blood. He mentioned similar findings in the blood of a psychopath who took many acetophenetidin tablets per day.

Cyanosis and altered blood pigments, particularly methemoglobin and sulfhemoglobin, were fairly common in early reports in patients who had taken large quantities of the drug for long periods of time. From the beginning it became obvious that very large doses of acetophenetidin were required to produce significant amounts of altered pigments. Experimentally in animals substantial doses of the drug are required to produce significant amounts of methemoglobin or sulfhemoglobin. After the discontinuance of the drug the methemoglobin disappears rapidly and the sulfhemoglobin somewhat more slowly. It appears probable that *N*-acetyl-*p*-aminophenol, even in large doses, is less apt to bring about the production of methemoglobin and sulfhemoglobin.

Effect on Leucocytes

Mahnert (307) stated that one of the effects of giving mammals large doses of acetophenetidin was that the white blood cells did not show typical amoeba-like movements. Krönig (256) recorded a considerable increase in the white blood cell count of a 17-year-old printer's apprentice who had taken 1-g. doses of acetophenetidin. When the patient came to autopsy it was noted, among other points, that he had chronic otitis media. The author assumed that the patient had been weakened by infection before he took the acetophenetidin which he normally tolerated well. Krönig (258) gave additional details on cases he had already published concerning the blood picture in cases of acetophenetidin poisoning. He wrote that the white cells were found in various stages of degeneration. Storozhevoj (469) observed a leucocyte count of 10,600 per mm.^{3} in a 16-year-old girl who had taken 25 g. of acetophenetidin with suicidal intent. On the sixth day the patient recovered and left the hospital with a leucocyte count of 4000 per mm.^{3} Poljakov (383) described the changes in leucocyte count in a university student who took 60 g. of acetophenetidin during 5 hours. Upon admission his white count was 7740 per mm.^{3} The third day his leucocyte count was 6340 per mm.^{3}, and the fifth day it was down to 4400 per mm.^{3} On the eleventh day there was a sharp rise to 36,680 per mm.^{3}, and on the twelfth day it was still up to 15,335 per mm.^{3} By the seventeenth day the count had dropped to 7740 per mm.^{3} The differential count did not change as much. The polynuclear cells were 78 per cent on the second day, fell to 40 per cent on the sixth day, and rose to 82 per cent on the eleventh day. The mononuclear cells rose from 20 per cent on the second day to 42 per cent on the sixth day, and fell to 15 per cent on the eleventh day. The eosinophiles were 0.5 per cent on the second day, 7.5 per cent on the sixth day, and back to 1 per cent on the eleventh day.

Reid (390) reported the case of a 28-year-old woman who had been taking acetophenetidin in large amounts for about 5 months. A leucocyte count revealed 7350 cells with 82 per cent neutrophiles, 10 per cent lymphocytes, 2.5 per cent endothelial cells, and 2.0 per cent basophiles. He did not record the leucocyte count at any other time. Kracke (248) indicated acetophenetidin (listed in the article as "phenacatine") as one of the drugs that had been taken by patients who later developed an agranulocytosis. He said that in 9 cases of agranulocytosis 8 had been taking either acetophenetidin, aminopyrine, peralga, or diallylbarbituric acid. He gave a rabbit 0.13 to 0.25 g. of acetophenetidin daily by oral administration for 45 days and found no effect on the leucocyte count. Fisher (131) listed a case of a 47-year-old man who had been taking large quantities of acetophenetidin and acetanilid over a long period of time and who, upon admission, had a leucocyte count of 12,000 per mm.[3] He gave no further data.

Costen (85) referred to the case of a 64-year-old woman who had taken large doses of aspirin, acetophenetidin, and bromides. Her leucocyte count was 1840 with 50 per cent granulocytes and this, plus the appearance of a pharyngeal lesion, suggested a diagnosis of agranulocytosis. This patient was recovering from a fractured femur. A physician advised X-irradiation of the long bone, the cast being opened to admit radiation. The temperature subsided, the pharynx became free of inflammation, and the blood counts returned to normal. She was discharged with a white count of 9600 per mm.[3] and 70 per cent granular cells. For 1 month she was free of symptoms, and the leucocyte count remained within the normal limits. She re-entered the hospital with a white count of 2600 per mm.[3] and a sloughing necrosis with gangrene of the pharynx. Daily radiation of the long bones was given with no apparent response; the white cell count dropped to 200 and she expired. The author concluded that regular ingestion of the drug for a long period of time was the chief factor in the depression of bone marrow function. He did not consider the repeated radiation to be a factor, despite the knowledge of the effects of such exposure.

Madison and Squier (305) discussed aminopyrine in relation to agranulocytosis but included a few records which suggested that acetanilid, acetophenetidin, dinitrophenol, and other drugs also might be of etiological importance. They stated that "the opportunity to prove the ability of any of these latter drugs to depress the granulocytes has not yet arisen." Madison and Squier (306) summarized 14 cases of primary granulocytopenia, showing the relationship of drugs containing aminopyrine to the onset and outcome of the disease. One of those mentioned concerned a 48-year-old housewife who took a mixture containing aminopyrine, acetophenetidin, caffeine, and hyoscyamus. Her white count was 1100 per mm.[3] with no granulocytes. The administration of barbiturates and aminopyrine continued, but she recovered in 8 months and there had been no recurrence of the disturbance. Kracke and Parker (250) recorded the case of a dentist with an acute fulminating form of the disease accompanied by complete loss of granulocytes. He had taken large doses of acetophenetidin, and the authors felt that this drug was incriminated along with aminopyrine in the production of the disease. They injected rabbits intraperitoneally with 0.3 g. of acetophenetidin per day for 60 days but found no depression of the leucocyte count. Similar negative results were obtained with 6 other drugs including aminopyrine. Kracke and Parker (251) described a middle-aged white man who had been taking 1 g. of aminopyrine daily and who was treated for mild influenza with capsules containing acetophenetidin just before the clinical onset of agranulocytosis. Also, they discussed the case of a middle-aged white woman who received 3 doses of neoarsphenamine and who in addition took a mixture containing acetophenetidin which had been prescribed by her dentist. Another middle-aged white woman had been given acetophenetidin for 5 years preceding the onset of her illness and during this period had taken so much of the drug that when she was admitted to the hospital with granulocytopenia she had the marked gray-blue color associated with sulfhemoglobinemia. Squier and Madison (463,464) discussed granulocytopenia due to aminopyrine. They gave no original data, but in a discussion of their paper Dr. Marion Sulzberger mentioned that "Dr. J. Wolf of New York recently called to my attention the fact that drugs which cause granulocytopenias are just those which cause fixed drug eruptions, e.g., the . . . phenacetin, amidopyrine; these are the main offenders in both conditions."

Kracke's hypothesis that agranulocytosis is caused by a common drug degradation product is questioned by Squier and Madison (464) who state that they failed to observe the phenomenon after the use of acetophenetidin in some of their patients. Kracke (249), in discussing the relation of drug therapy to neutropenic states, mentioned that acetophenetidin had been named in two cases by Kracke and Parker (251) and in one case by Costen (85).

Lundsteen *et al.* (293,294) found, in a 62-year-old man who had taken large amounts of acetophenetidin for at least 13 months, a white cell count of 11,100 per $mm.^3$ with 76 per cent polynuclear neutrophiles, 2 per cent eosinophiles, 1 per cent basophiles, 4 per cent monocytes, and 17 per cent lymphocytes. They gave no further data on the leucocytes. In 1936 Kracke and Parker (253) related acetophenetidin to the leucopenic state by their observations of a white woman with a leucocyte count of 500 and with a severe methemoglobinemia said to be due to the long continued use of acetophenetidin. In reviewing 187 published cases they noted that acetophenetidin had been administered in 2 of them. Hammarsten and Nordenfelt (178) observed a white cell count of 7900 per mm.^{3} with 52 per cent neutrophiles, 0 per cent eosinophiles, 3 per cent lymphocytes, and 13 per cent monocytes in a 46-year-old woman who for 7 years had taken a mixture containing acetophenetidin.

Adams *et al.* (1) studied the effects of prolonged daily administration of acetophenetidin in 2 series of 6 dogs. After several weeks of control study, 4 dogs in each series were given daily doses of 15 mg. of acetophenetidin per kg. for 3 months. The total and differential leucocyte counts were within the normal limits of the variations noted in control animals and in each animal's own control period.

Jasinski and Müller (231) referred to a patient who exhibited the chronic effects of an acetophenetidin mixture. Upon admission the leucocyte count was 4400 per mm.^{3} with 63 per cent segmented, 10.5 per cent monocytes, and 20 per cent lymphocytes. Eight days later the leucocyte count was 6100 per mm.^{3} with 64 per cent segmented, 6.5 per cent monocytes, and 21 per cent lymphocytes. They also reported the case of a 54-year-old housewife who had been taking this mixture daily and had a leucocyte count of 11,000 per mm.,^{3} and of a 47-year-old housewife taking the same drug who had a leucocyte count of 14,300 per mm.^{3} Merlevede (325) describes a 51-year-old woman who had been taking the mixture in large doses for a long period of time and who upon examination had a white count of 7200 per mm.^{3} as well as the case of a 39-year-old woman who had been taking powders containing acetophenetidin, antipyrine, and caffeine for a long period of time with a resulting white count of 4300 per mm.^{3}

Recent textbooks (449) conclude that "there is no evidence of depression of bone marrow activity after administration of therapeutic doses of acetanilid, acetophenetidin, or *N*-acetyl-*p*-aminophenol," and Goodman and Gilman (160) conclude that neither acetanilid nor acetophenetidin cause agranulocytosis.

N-Acetyl-p-aminophenol. Killian (241) gave 62 human subjects 0.8 g. of *N*-acetyl-*p*-aminophenol daily for 24 to 56 days without observable adverse effects. There were no blood changes in 25 of the subjects studied. Conklin (82) gave *N*-acetyl-*p*-aminophenol to patients in doses up to 6 g. per day for anywhere from 6 weeks to 1 year without adverse effects. Remsen (392) described 3 patients who had low leucocyte counts while receiving a mixture of *N*-acetyl-*p*-aminophenol, aspirin, and caffeine. In one the leucocyte count fell from 4400 to 1600 per mm.^{3}, in another it fell from 7100 to 625 per mm.^{3}, and in the third from 5500 to 850 per mm.^{3} All were receiving other drugs at the same time and all regained normal leucocyte counts while under observation. Rovenstine (405) found no change in the complete blood count of 10 patients receiving 0.17 g. of *N*-acetyl-*p*-aminophenol four times a day for 10 days. Doses of 3.6 g. *N*-acetyl-*p*-aminophenol daily for as long as 116 weeks produced no blood disturbances (25). Kracke and Parker (252) reviewed the evidence as to whether certain drugs cause agranulocytosis. They concluded : "It is questionable as to whether acetanilid, acetophenetidine, antipyrine, acetylsalicylic acid and quinine are capable of producing the disease."

Early reports associating diminished leucocyte counts with the administration of drugs sometimes mentioned acetophenetidin along with the others. There is no evidence that even when patients were given large doses of acetophenetidin for long periods of time, there was any significant depression of the leucocyte count. Certain reports of the occurrence of low leucocyte counts during or following the administration of acetophenetidin or of *N*-acetyl-*p*-aminophenol have been criticized as perhaps not excluding the effect of other factors.

It may be observed that there is no demonstrated relationship between the ingestion of acetophenetidin and the leucocyte count.

Effects on Respiration

Forschelen (135) observed that when the drug was given to patients with fever they showed a decrease in respiratory rate. The greater the initial number of respirations per minute the greater was the decrease in rate. Lackie (262) reported the case of a patient given acetophenetidin at the rate of 0.7 g. every 4 hours at first, then 1.0 g. every 4 hours, and finally, because of severe pain, 1.0 g. every 2 hours. Within a few minutes the patient complained of shortness of breath, which was so marked that he had to sit up in bed, and of restlessness which compelled him to walk around the room constantly gasping for breath. On two subsequent occasions the patient repeated the 1.0-g. dose at short intervals with the same accompanying symptoms. The attacks continued for about 15 min. and then subsided. Another case was reported in which the details were obtained by correspondence with a medical friend who, suffering from influenza, had taken 1.3 g. of the drug every 2 hours for 6 doses. This resulted in dyspnea resembling that seen in other patients. The symptoms continued for 1 hour after which his friend continued the drug with no further toxic effects.

Löbl (285) described a case of a law student who took 1 g. of acetophenetidin and suffered severe toxic effects. He was seen about an hour after taking the second 0.5-g. powder and had difficulty in breathing. Upon examination the respiration was found to be shallow and the rate was 24 per min. with an occasional noisy inspiration.

Poljakov (383) recorded a case of a patient who took 60 g. of acetophenetidin during a 5 hour period, and it was observed that there was no respiratory distress. Reid (390) described a case of a 28-year-old woman who reported that she had taken large amounts of acetophenetidin for about 5 months. Among other symptoms was a rapid shallow respiration at a rate of 70 to 80 per min. It was determined later, however, that the rapid respiratory rate was of nervous origin since it returned to normal when the patient was asleep and unaware of observation.

Hare (182) gave 65 mg. of acetophenetidin to an 85-g. frog and reported that it died of respiratory failure since the heart continued to give an occasional abortive beat.

Ledoux (267) administered acetophenetidin subcutaneously, intravenously, or orally to guinea pigs, rabbits, white mice, and dogs, and reported that large doses caused marked dyspnea and then the animals stopped breathing. He suggested that the drug paralyzed the respiratory center.

Mahnert (307) observed that when rabbits were given large doses of the drug (1.5 g to an 870-g. rabbit and 4.5 g. to a 750-g. rabbit) there was an increase in respiratory rate followed by cessation of respiration. Hambourger (175) gave very large doses of acetophenetidin to rabbits and, among other symptoms, noted a slow deep respiration with occasional sneezing and dripping of clear fluid from the nose.

Dreser (99) found that when he gave 0.2 g. of acetophenetidin to a cat with a normal respiratory capacity of 17.2 per cent this had decreased to 8.2 per cent by the next day. When he gave 0.1 g. there was no change. When he gave 0.1 g. acetanilid, the respiratory capacity fell from 14.0 per cent to 6.1 per cent.

Hinsberg and Kast (206) gave dogs weighing 5 to 6 kg., 1 to 2 g. of acetophenetidin a day for several days and later increased the dose to 3 to 5 g. a day; they observed an acceleration in respiratory rate. Cerna and Carter (70) observed that after intravenous doses of several grams of acetophenetidin in dogs there was a progressive fall in blood pressure, the respiratory rate also decreased, and the respiration ceased before the heart stopped. Wood and Wood (524) injected the drug suspended in 0.7 per cent salt solution into the jugular vein of a dog. Doses of 0.5 g. per kg. caused death from respiratory failure.

N-Acetyl-p-aminophenol. Hinsberg and Treupel (207) gave 7 g. of *N*-acetyl-*p*-aminophenol intravenously in small doses to a female rabbit weighing 1950 g. After 3 hours following a dose of 4 g., the respiratory rate rose from 33 to 57 per min. After a dosage of 7 g., 4 hours and 10 min. later the respiration stopped.

Summary. Neither in the human nor in experimental animals is there evidence that moderate doses of acetophenetidin or *N*-acetyl-*p*-aminophenol produce any significant effects upon the respiratory system.

Effect on Renal Function

Clinical Observations

The early reports of the use of acetophenetidin rarely mentioned the effects of the drug on renal function. Köbler (245) reported that acetophenetidin had no undesirable effects in patients with nephritis. There was no evidence of increased protein excretion. No impairment of renal function in the human was observed by Hare (182) after moderate doses were employed for the relief of pain.

In some cases where patients have received large doses of acetophenetidin, usually for long periods of time, there are some reports claiming renal damage. It is not evident that acetophenetidin was the causative agent.

Cattani (68) twice observed hematuria and nephritis in patients receiving acetophenetidin, and Rifat (397) observed uremia and oliguria in a 65-year-old woman who had been taking 5 g. of acetophenetidin per day, but it is not clear that the findings were related to drug administration. Krönig (256) described a patient, presumably suffering from lead poisoning, who took acetophenetidin in 1-g.

doses. He became quite ill with headaches, vomiting, and diarrhea. The patient became yellow and died shortly thereafter. Post mortem examination revealed kidneys large and noticeably brown. Urine removed from the bladder by means of a catheter was thick and dark brown-red in color but it contained no white corpuscles. It is not known if the patient suffered from a liver disease. Meurice (327,328) discussed a case of a woman who took 11 g. of acetophenetidin within 20 hours. He remarked on the fact that at no time was there any evidence of renal damage. Russow (407) cited the case of a woman who had taken moderate doses of acetophenetidin for the relief of intense pain which began after lightning had struck near her. She was given several drugs, including morphine. She became unconscious, quite cyanotic, and died. Upon examination of the urine, which was collected by means of a catheter, it was found to be dark brown in color and gave a reaction for methemoglobin. It also contained large numbers of urinary cylinders covered with fine amorphous gray-brown spots. Poljakov (383) related a case of a young man who took 60 g. of acetophenetidin during 5 hours. At first the urine was quite normal but by the sixth day it showed all signs of nephritis including 6 per cent albumin, granular cylinders, cells of kidney epithelia, red blood corpuscles, and leucocytes. During the next 36 hours the leucocytes disappeared from the urine and only traces of signs of nephritis remained, including an insignificant amount of albumin which, however, was still detectable in the urine after 19 days.

Thölen (477) observed that 2 patients who gave a history of chronic administration of a mixture containing 250 mg. acetophenetidin, 150 mg. isopropylantipyrine, 50 mg. Persedon, and 50 mg. caffeine had chronic interstitial nephritis, but there was little evidence the condition was due to the drug. In 40 cases of chronic ingestion of acetophenetidin-containing preparations that Schweingruber (426) studied, he observed renal symptoms in 47 per cent and urea retention in 32 per cent. Spühler and Zollinger (462) studied a number of cases of chronic interstitial nephritis, 7 of which had taken for a number of years this same mixture containing acetophenetidin, caffeine, isopropylantipyrine, and Persedon. They were not able to say whether the drug administration was associated with the renal pathology. Later Zollinger (529) reported that, of 62 patients with chronic interstitial nephritis, 18 had been taking the mixture for 1.5 to 22 years. This same mixture is mentioned as being associated in 8 or 9 cases of interstitial nephritis with tubular damage described by Moeschlin (337). It should be noted that little is known about the possible role of isopropylantipyrine and Persedon in the nephritis described and one should reserve judgment in attributing it to acetophenetidin until this drug alone is shown to be responsible. More recently Thölen and co-workers (478) have expressed the opinion that the chronic administration of this mixture decreased or inactivated the renal carbonic anhydrase with a resultant acidosis leading to renal damage.

Experimental Observations

Rats. Martin (317) observed an increase in urinary uric acid elimination in rats after 500 mg. per kg. but no effect upon allantoin elimination. Hasegawa and Pfeiffer (190) found that acetophenetidin, given orally twice daily in doses of 100 mg., decreased but did not abolish the glycosuria of alloxan diabetic rats. Studer and Zbinden (472) attempted to contribute to the problem of renal damage after the administration of analgesic drugs. They gave rats either 60 mg. per kg. of 3,3-diethyl-2,4-dioxotetrahydropyridine, 300 mg. per kg. of acetophenetidin, 180 mg. per kg. of 1-phenyl-2,3-dimethyl-4-isopropyl-5-pyrazolone, 60 mg. per kg. of caffeine, or a mixture of all the aforementioned. The rats weighed 90 to 98 g. each at the beginning of the experiment. Groups of 10 were given the preceding doses 5 days a week for 6.5 months. At autopsy the animals had normal blood morphology and no demonstrable abnormalities of the kidneys.

Rabbits. Morinaka (340) gave one rabbit 4.75 g. of acetophenetidin and determined the composition of the urine before, during, and after administration. The renal excretion of nitrogen changed very slightly. There was no change in excretion of ammonia nitrogen and only a very slight rise in the amino acid nitrogen compared to the total nitrogen. The author concluded that acetophenetidin had a destructive effect on protein which he felt might be related to a functional disturbance of cell protoplasm by the drug. Averbuck (16) gave rabbits 400 mg. of acetophenetidin per kg. orally and observed 50 per cent inhibition of diuresis in 4 out of the 5 animals and 30 per cent in the other one. The excretion of sodium chloride was not appreciably affected. Liaci (278) found that acetophenetidin, given orally to dogs in doses of 0.75 g. per day and to rabbits in doses of 500 mg. per kg. did not interfere with intestinal absorption of nitrogen-containing substances. The urine volume was the same, and its reaction remained acidic. Phosphate excretion and chloride excretion were increased. Total sulfate and combined sulfates decreased, total nitrogen and urea excretion increased. Griffi (166) gave a dog 0.75 g. of acetophenetidin and observed the urinary elimination of various substances over the next 11 days. Lagutin (263) studied the effects of acetophenetidin on the blood pressure of rabbits perfused with a 1:2000 solution of the drug. There was an abrupt moderate decrease followed by fairly rapid return to normal. The vessels of the kidney changed a little in their diameter but probably not from a direct effect upon their contraction. Other experiments suggested that the decrease in the size of the kidney was due mainly to the lesser blood flow into the organ because of the sharp fall in the blood pressure.

Cats. In experiments on cats with oncometers on the kidney and back leg, Lagutin (263) observed that the decrease in kidney size could be accounted for by the decrease in blood pressure.

Dogs. Pitini and Hamnett (379) gave a 5.27-kg. dog, 0.25 g. of acetophenetidin and observed a moderate increase in urea, phosphorus, and sodium chloride excretion. Adams *et al.* (1) studied the effect of prolonged daily administration of 15 mg. acetophenetidin per kg., which corresponded to the therapeutic dose in man, in 2 series of 6 dogs each. They performed kidney function tests for several weeks and observed no changes at any time.

Effects on the Liver

Clinical Observations

In the 23-year-old patient who had taken 60 g. of acetophenetidin, Poljakov (383) found that the liver was both enlarged and quite sensitive to the touch, at first, but that it became less sensitive by the sixth day. During most of this interval the enlargement of the liver persisted accompanied by severe jaundice, and the size of the organ approached normal only after 9 days.

Even when the clinical signs of acetophenetidin intoxication such as cyanosis and anemia were evident, Wuhrmann and Jasinski (525) found the size of the liver and spleen to be normal.

Experimental Observations

Mice. Because some compounds related to aniline had been shown to produce liver tumors in mice, Schmähl and Reiter (420) studied acetophenetidin and obtained evidence that it was not carcinogenic.

Rats. In experiments to elucidate the effects on carbohydrate metabolism, normal male albino rats, weighing between 150 to 290 g., were fasted overnight and 4 hours before sacrifice, were given 5 ml. per kg. of 40 per cent glucose solution intraperitoneally, and two hours before sacrifice were given 4 millimoles of acetophenetidin per kg. plus 4 millimoles of sodium bicarbonate. The terminal blood glucose was 129 mg. per 100 ml. compared with 125 mg. per 100 ml. in the control animals given saline solutions (127). The liver glycogen of the animals given the glucose solution and acetophenetidin was 2.77 per cent of the fresh tissue which was slightly higher than the value of 2.53 per cent in the saline controls. The muscle glycogen of the former group was only 0.50 per cent in the fresh tissue compared with 1.31 per cent in the control animals. A similar dose of acetophenetidin resulted in diminished concentrations of ascorbic acid in the adrenals. The animals receiving the drug had an average concentration of 0.210 per cent compared with 0.376 per cent in the controls (127).

Dogs. Acetophenetidin, in small doses, did not have any effect on the secretion of the gall bladder of bile fistula dogs, but medium sized doses increased the volume and dilution of the bile secreted. The absolute content of solids was within normal limits but was less than the normal average. Both dogs received 0.2 g. of acetophenetidin per dose, one dog getting it two and three times a day and the other dog getting it four times a day (517). Adams *et al.* (1) studied the effect of prolonged daily administration of 15 mg. of acetophenetidin per kg. to dogs for 3 months and found that it had no effect upon liver function.

Effects on the Spleen

The spleen of the 17-year-old printer's apprentice who took 4 doses of 1 gram of acetophenetidin over a 3 week period was enlarged, of normal consistency, and easily palpable (256). He died and at autopsy the spleen was found to be enlarged, of rough consistency, and dark brown in color. It was probable he suffered from lead poisoning. Poljakov (383) observed that on the fourth day after a student had taken 60 g. of acetophenetidin, the spleen was enlarged, but 3 days later it was near normal size. Jasinski (231) found that in a 20-year-old girl who took 20 to 30 tablets of acetophenetidin a day, the spleen was easily felt. Cerny (71) observed that in a 1-month old child who had been given relatively large doses of acetophenetidin by suppository, the spleen could be felt $1^1/_2$ finger widths below the costal margin. Within 2 weeks she had improved greatly, and the spleen was no longer palpable. He reported a similar finding on a 2-month-old girl and a 4-month-old boy who has been given suppositories containing acetophenetidin. A woman, who had taken large doses of acetophenetidin for a long period of time, was said to have had an enlarged spleen (427).

Brownlee (53) gave 25 per cent of the LD_{50} of actophenetidin daily to rats. Upon histological examination the spleens were grossly abnormal, enlarged and blue-black in color. The sinuses were engorged and quantities of stainable iron were seen. In the pulp there were considerable deposits of brownish nonstaining pigment.

Effect on the Adrenals

Large doses of acetophenetidin (4 mM. per kg.) produced a marked depletion of the ascorbic acid of the adrenals of rats (127). Similar results were obtained by Noach *et al.* (354) who gave the drug daily. They observed no depletion of adrenal cholesterol.

General Effects on Metabolism

Frogs. Mandewirth (312) measured the oxygen consumption of various tissues in the presence of acetophenetidin and related drugs. The oxygen uptake of the frog skeletal muscle was depressed measurably by 10^{-6} molar concentrations of acetophenetidin, and as much as 50 per cent by 10^{-4} molar.

Rats. Brownlee (53) gave groups of adult male rats 25 per cent of the LD_{50} of acetophenetidin and alternated periods of treatment with intervals when the animals received no drug. The animals showed poor appetites and lost weight during the periods of acetophenetidin administration.

Svirbely (474) studied the effect of acetophenetidin in young albino rats maintained on a diet devoid of ascorbic acid. Four female albino rats were given 160 mg. of acetophenetidin mixed with 10 g. of diet daily for a period of 31 days. The initial average weight of the animals was 142 g. and their final average weight when they were destroyed at the age of 98 days was 152 g. In the treated group the total ascorbic acid content of various organs was found to be: adrenals, 0.02 mg.; liver, 0.65 mg.; small intestine, 0.84 mg.; and spleen, 0.10 mg. The corresponding values for the controls were, respectively, 0.06 mg., 0.61 mg., 0.75 mg., and 0.10 mg. The concentration of ascorbic acid in the adrenals was only 0.71 mg. per g. in the animals getting acetophenetidin as compared with 1.84 mg. per g. in the controls. A similar decrease in adrenal ascorbic acid was observed after acetanilid and to a smaller extent after aminopyrine administration.

Rakieten (389) demonstrated that in rats 200 mg. of acetophenetidin per kg. did not lower the rate at which ethyl alcohol disappeared from the blood. However larger doses given 1 hour before the alcohol was administered reduced the rate of disappearance to less than $^{1}/_{2}$ of that found in the control animals. When these same doses were given 40 hours before the alcohol, the rate of disappearance was within the normal range.

Acetophenetidin in a dose of 4.0 millimoles per kg. had no effect on the blood glucose or liver glycogen concentrations of rats but it did result in much lower concentrations of muscle glycogen (127).

Rabbits and cats. With acetophenetidin, Mandewirth (312) observed a definite decrease in the oxygen consumption of rabbit heart muscle in the presence of 1 per cent sodium lactate, and of cat skeletal muscle which had been washed three times to remove most of the enzymes and substrates. He believed that the amount of drug required to reduce oxygen consumption was comparable to an amount constituting a reasonable dose in man and he therefore concluded that the action of the drug might be explained through some such mechanism. Horigeshi (217) administered the drug to rabbits and studied various effects.

Dogs. In attempts to determine the mode of action of acetophenetidin in dogs with fever produced experimentally, Cerna and Carter (70) used a calorimeter and concluded that the drug reduced heat production but did not increase heat dissipation. Piccinini (375) gave dogs doses of 100 to 236 mg. actophenetidin per kg. and observed that the oxygen consumption usually decreased as did the carbon dioxide production.

Piccinini (373) gave large doses of acetophenetidin orally to dogs and found that the viscosity of the serum was increased.

Sakanian (410) studied the effects of acetophenetidin on the reflex secretion of the stomach.

Human. Livierato (284) used normal subjects and determined their basal metabolic rate after acetophenetidin and other antipyretics. The diminution in carbon dioxide production was more marked after acetophenetidin than after acetanilid. The excretion of urea fluctuated but tended to increase somewhat. Generally the urinary secretion was decreased during the administration of acetophenetidin, particularly during the first days. The amount of carbon dioxide excreted decreased progressively with administration of the drug.

Sokolov (455) observed that, among children given acetophenetidin, there was increased evaporation through the skin in female patients which would start $^1/_2$ to 1 hour after intake; sweating, however, was excessive only in very rare exceptions.

Baccarani (20) observed that, in two patients without fever on a normal diet, acetophenetidin increased the excretion of ethereal sulfate.

When two human subjects were given 1.3 g. of acetophenetidin with 120 ml. 90-proof whiskey, the drug did not have any effect on the rate of disappearance of alcohol from the blood (389). This suggested that, whatever effects the drug had, they were exercised through its action on the liver.

Effect on Enzyme Systems

Georgievsky (151) prepared artificial gastric juice and added to it acetophenetidin in alcohol coagulated egg albumin. When he placed the mixture in an air bath at 35 to 40°C., there was no inhibition of protein digestion. In experiments to test the effects of acetophenetidin on alcoholic fermentation, it was shown that the quantity of carbon dioxide produced was appreciably greater when acetophenetidin was added.

Burge (57) determined the effect of acetophenetidin on the production of catalase by the liver, using tissue removed from rabbits and dogs under ether anesthesia. The catalase content of jugular vein blood from animals given acetophenetidin also was determined. Acetophenetidin had no effect on the catalase of the blood either *in vivo* or *in vitro*. Although there was a slight increase in catalase production by the liver, this was not great enough to account for the effect of acetophenetidin in lowering the body temperature. Vegter (496) studied the anticatalase action of several drugs, including acetophenetidin, which he found was very active in this respect, much more so than either salicylic acid or acetanilid.

Michel *et al.* (330) studied the effect of acetophenetidin upon the acylases which they prepared from ground rat liver by acetone extraction. If the hydrolysis rate of acetanilid was assigned a value of 100, the relative hydrolysis rate of acetophenetidin was no more than approximately 14. This low rate may have been due to the relative insolubility of acetophenetidin in the reaction medium.

Boutaric and Gauthier (42) found that acetophenetidin as well as some other analgesic drugs decreased slightly the time required for a hog liver homogenate to decolorize methylene blue. It was their suggestion that the mechanism of action of analgesic drugs might be connected with the antioxygen action. They also suggested that the antipyretic action is related to this. Michelson (331) compared the action of acetophenetidin and several other drugs upon the activity of choline esterase, using concentrations of the drugs which were equal in their narcotic effect on frogs. Acetophenetidin in a molar concentration of 2.8×10^{-3} produced an appreciable inhibition.

Horikawa (218) found that acetophenetidin had no effect upon the activity of thiaminase in human feces.

Preparations of the acid phosphatase of dog liver studied by Bertran and Sanchez (31) were found to be activated by as much as 50 per cent by the addition of acetophenetidin at a concentration of 1:1000.

A pyruvate decarboxylase from fetuses and the tissues of young rabbits is inhibited by acetophenetidin as well as by several other analgesic drugs (413).

In a recent significant study devoted primarily to elucidating the mechanism of action of salicylates Brody (50) found that 2×10^{-3} molar acetophenetidin had a weak effect or none on the uncoupling of oxidative phosphorylation. The enzyme was prepared from rat liver mitochondria. Salicylates, on the other hand, were very potent as uncouplers. So far the small amount of experimental data on the effects of acetophenetidin on enzyme systems has not clarified the mechanism of the action.

Other Effects

Horigeshi (217) recorded simultaneously the movements of the uterus and the intestinal canal of rabbits that had been injected with small doses of acetophenetidin. No changes were observed.

Chapter X

Toxicology

Clinical Observations

It is not surprising that the large doses of acetophenetidin so commonly used when the drug was introduced led occasionally to untoward effects. Later when it became generally available, especially in mixtures with other drugs, there were further instances in which toxic effects occurred, usually after the prolonged use of large doses. Often it is very difficult to separate the effects of acetophenetidin from those of other drugs given concurrently.

Robertson (399) objected to the indiscriminate use of antipyretics and pointed out that they might produce harmful effects in patients. In an early anonymous article (11) it was pointed out that acetophenetidin might be substituted in proprietary mixtures for acetanilid but that there was no evidence that it was less harmful. In an editorial (112) entitled "The harmful effects of acetanilid, antipyrine and phenacetin," the effects of acetanilid are mentioned but there is no discussion of acetophenetidin.

Effects on Skin

It is interesting to note that in the older literature there are frequent references to skin disorders due to administration of acetophenetidin. Hoppe (215) mentions a 22-year-old male with typhoid fever, who, after a dose of 0.5 g. of acetophenetidin, noticed an exanthema similar to that produced by quinine or antipyrine. The second dose produced a reddening of the skin, with itching and reddening on the arms and upper thighs. The following day the exanthema remained but there was less itching. The probability of a rash due to the disease was not discussed. Valentin (494) lists the case of a woman with anemia and headaches who, for two successive evenings after she had received 0.6 g. of the drug, felt great heat in the face and therefore could not sleep. Her husband noticed that her whole body, but especially the arms and legs, was covered with red spots. The lesions were about the size of a pea and appeared pointed with the center darker than the outside. Other lesions were flat and became pale with pressure. There was no pain or itching on the body. The exanthema disappeared completely by the following day, but the patient was without appetite and had a feeling of tiredness. The author believed that this was a case exhibiting an idiosyncrasy. Hirschfelder (209) observed 3 or 4 patients who complained of an exanthema with considerable burning pain, which usually disappeared by the following day. Öffinger (356) recorded the case of a patient who had suffered severe pain for 2 years. He was given 1 g. of acetophenetidin every 3 hours. The patient reported relief from his sciatic pain but one morning observed edema under both lower eyelids. With continued use of the drug the edematous swelling of the eyelids, the forehead, the nose, and the upper part of the cheek were noted to resemble the facial edema seen during nephritis. There also was swelling of all the fingers so that it was impossible to move the joints. At a later date, the patient was given a "challenging trial" with 4 doses of 0.5 g. of the drug and the symptoms recurred. It would appear that this patient exhibited an allergic reaction to the drug. Horváth (219, 220) reported that one of the undesirable side-effects was occasional sweating. Two cases exhibited dermatitis which disappeared when the substance was discontinued. One typhus patient who had received 0.12 to 0.25 g. of the drug for 6 days exhibited a rash on the left shoulder, both elbows, and on the back of the left hand. The rash consisted of small bumps slightly raised above the surface of the skin; some were isolated and some coalesced and tended to blanch under pressure. The patient did not complain of itching or pain. The rash disappeared completely within 3 days. Apparently a rash due to the disease was not considered. Another patient, after 0.5 to 1.5 g. of acetophenetidin daily for 30 days for neuralgia developed an itching rash, qualitatively similar to the one described in the foregoing. The rash was upon the extremities, the back, and the middle of the chest. Three days after discontinuing the drug, the itching ceased. In reviewing the untoward effects of acetophenetidin and some other analgesic drugs, Paterson (367) mentioned that skin eruptions, chiefly urticarias, were produced. West (512) reported a case in which two 0.7-g. doses of the drug at 4-hour intervals caused a measly rash on the face, trunk, and extremities. A 28-year-old man, 3 hours after taking 0.3-g. tablets, is said to have become covered by a scarletinoform rash accompanied by a slight tingling sensation.

Two hours after its onset, the rash disappeared and the patient had no further complaints. Subsequent administration of the drug in 0.3- to 1.0-g. doses caused a recurrence of the rash which varied in intensity according to the dose. This case was most likely due to an idiosyncrasy (513). Another case was that of a young woman with facial neuralgia, who, 1 to 2 hours after taking 0.3- to 1.0-g. doses, exhibited an urticarial rash with raised wheals on the face and neck. The rash was accompanied by a tingling sensation which lasted a couple of hours. Kibbe (239) reported the case of a 50-year-old woman who had ecchymotic spots and pruritus which were attributed to acetophenetidin. She had taken the prescribed dose of 0.3 g. every 3 hours for 6 doses. The following day she complained of itching of the skin over the abdomen and limbs which was relieved by the use of alcohol and salt water. When she returned to the clinic on the fourth day, large ecchymotic areas were seen on the inner side of each thigh near the groin as well as smaller ones scattered over the abdomen and the limbs. The lesions gradually faded out. No other symptoms were reported. Hirschfeld (208) cited the case of a patient, a 23-year-old woman, who had had a skin rash for 2 months. The lower thighs were well covered with a longitudinal and pointed petechiae. On the lower half of the tibia there were slight hemorrhages. The center of the lesions were ulcerated and painful to the touch. They were about 2 or 3 mm. deep. There was no apparent cause for the ulcers and she had no idea as to what had started them. Treatment with potassium iodide was unsuccessful. It occurred to the physician that this condition might be associated with the ingestion of acetophenetidin which the patient used for the relief of migraine. When the drug was discontinued the general condition of the patient improved. The petechiae became pale, leaving behind a brown pigment, and the ulcers closed. In order to confirm the diagnosis, the patient again was given acetophenetidin and after 1.5 g. per week it was reported that new hemorrhages and a new ulcer were observed. A 48-year-old woman reported to have taken 11 g. of the drug within 24 hours also developed an erythema; the spots were darker in the center than in the periphery and they blanched out under pressure (327,328). Blisters of the same color also were observed. The erythema had subsided in less than 1 day. A 22-year-old man took a single dose of 0.5 g. of antipyrine and the following day reported that he had had swollen eyelids and lips and an eruption on the scrotum (264). Sometime later he took 0.25 g. of acetophenetidin, and the following day skin eruptions, swollen eyelids and lips, and a strong albuminuria were observed. This patient was known to have had scarlet fever with some degree of albuminuria at the age of 17. Crohn (88), in a personal experiment, took a mixture of aminopyrine and a barbiturate; 2 years later he tried a mixture of aspirin, acetophenetidin, dimethylaminophenazone, diethylbarbituric acid, and caffeine. During each test Crohn developed urticaria of the extremities, edema of the penis and scrotum with reddening and itch. He also tested a mixture of sodium diethylbarbiturate, acetophenetidin, and codeine with the result that the following morning urticarial areas of varying sizes were observed upon the hand, upper thigh, and toes, together with edema of the penis and erythema of the scrotum. It is to be noted that all of these mixtures contained a barbiturate and two of them contained aminopyrine. Nevertheless Crohn assumed that since he had previously taken barbital and aminopyrine without side-effects, neither could be responsible for the results in these instances. He did not take acetophenetidin alone to prove whether it was capable of producing such lesions. A 62-year-old man, who during the preceding year had taken 1-g. acetophenetidin tablets at the rate of 4 a day, developed an extensive rash and severe headaches (294). At the time of hospitalization he exhibited a red punctate exanthema on the trunk and arms. Haxthausen (191) was the author of a paper concerning skin reactions after the administration of acetophenetidin but only the title is available in the literature. A review by Brown (51) states that acetophenetidin may cause skin reactions. He does not present any original data, therefore he probably referred to these poorly documented cases and to the few cases showing an idiosyncrasy.

Although skin disorders have been reported in patients given acetophenetidin, there is little evidence that these occur commonly. In most of the patients the evidence is not convincing that the administration of acetophenetidin was associated with the reported disturbances. Frequently acetophenetidin was given along with other drugs known to be more frequently associated with the production of untoward effects on the skin.

Nonfatal Toxic Effects in the Human

In 1890 Falk (123) summarized the various symptoms of toxicity which had been reported for acetophenetidin and reviewed much of the early work.

Harold (183) described the symptoms in a 32-year-old woman who had taken 3.3 to 5.3 g. of actophenetidin within 24 hours. She suddenly complained of a rapid pulse, headache, and shortness of breath. There were no urinary or gastric disturbances. Among other cases described by Knowles (244) was that of a woman who had taken 2 headache powders containing acetophenetidin and then later 0.6 g. of this drug itself. She had a slow pulse, difficult respiration, and general cyanosis but she recovered in 3 hours.

Meurice (327,328) described a 48-year-old woman who presumably had available 24 doses of acetophenetidin of 1 g. each, but the exact number that she took was not known. She suffered collapse, cyanosis, and cold extremities. After treatment with heat, caffeine, and sodium bicarbonate she improved gradually, although the cyanosis was still evident on the fourth day.

Kebler *et al.* (238) received 306 replies to 925 letters sent with test questionnaires to physicians concerning poisoning with acetanilid, antipyrine, and acetophenetidin. In the replies 95 cases of intoxication were attributed to acetophenetidin, as compared with 614 cases of intoxication attributed to acetanilid. The medical literature for the period covering 1884 to 1907 records 70 cases described as acetophenetidin poisoning, and, correspondingly, 297 cases attributed to acetanilid poisoning. More than 70 per cent of the cases reported as poisoning resulted from the prescription use of the drugs. This survey indicated that acetophenetidin was the most frequently used of all three drugs and that it was regarded as the least harmful.

In 1910 Boone (36) published the results of a questionnaire he had sent to a number of hospitals concerning untoward occurrences after the administration of antipyrine, acetanilid, and acetophenetidin. Thirty-one hospitals reported unfavorable results with either acetophenetidin or acetanilid, but there were no deaths recorded. He observed that in almost every instance where the drug had produced untoward results the dose had been larger than that generally recommended. He also noted that most of the unfavorable results occurred during the first years that the drugs were used. The one most frequently mentioned as causing symptoms was acetanilid, although frequently the drug used was not specified. Acetophenetidin was mentioned only in one case.

A patient of Welsford (509) through error took within the space of 1 hour about 5 g. of acetophenetidin and an hour later felt nauseated and depressed. Two hours later his temperature was below normal and his countenance was ash-gray and drawn. There was marked cyanosis, difficult respiration, and an irregular slow pulse. The principal symptoms disappeared within 3 hours but the next day he was still depressed and cyanotic. He had completely recovered by the following day.

In an analysis of 60 cases of reported drug intoxication in children, Murray (350) cites a single case due to acetophenetidin. This resulted from the administration of 0.2 g. of acetophenetidin in solution in 4 hours to a 2-month-old infant. The infant presented symptoms of collapse with cyanosis and a weak pulse.

Reissmann (391) discussed the toxicity of acetophenetidin in a 41-year-old woman, known to have been a morphine addict, who took a mixture of codeine and acetophenetidin regularly. During the first 3 years she took 10 tablets a day and then increased this to 20 tablets a day for the next 4 years. He estimated a daily intake of 5 g. In the 7 years, this patient consumed a total of 12 kg. of acetophenetidin.

Westhaus (514) attributed 3 cases of acute acetophenetidin intoxication in infants to the use of suppositories containing 0.125 g. acetophenetidin, 0.0625 g. aspirin, and 0.005 g. codeine phosphate. Two of the patients also appeared to be unduly depressed, presumably by the codeine.

Schaub *et al.* (416) reported that they had observed 24 cases of acetophenetidin intoxication during the preceding 3 years. These included 20 women and 4 men. In most cases the women were neurotic or psychopaths who had been using a mixture containing acetophenetidin for years. Some of them were said to have taken up to 12,000 tablets a year. All the patients showed cyanosis, and there was said to be evidence of sulfhemoglobinemia. Montero Rodríguez (339) observed a 1-year-old patient who became ill after receiving 150 mg. acetophenetidin, 200 mg. antipyrine, and 200 mg. aminopyrine. Clinical findings included somnolence, prostration, dilated pupils unreactive to light, lack of conjunctival reflexes, bradycardia, and symptoms of vascular collapse.

Schweingruber (426) discussed the problem of chronic intoxication after the administration of combinations of drugs containing acetophenetidin. Wuhrmann and Jasinski (525) considered 35 cases of toxic hemolytic anemia observed in patients following the administration of acetophenetidin. Of these, 32 were women and 3 were men. Fifteen cases were reviewed in some detail. They believed that the manifest form of acetophenetidin cyanosis was sex linked and that an iron deficiency, which is more common in women, probably was a prerequisite for the appearance of clinical manifestations. They believed that the toxic hemolytic anemia which developed was the result of disturbances in enzyme systems which detoxify and protect hemoglobin.

Allies (5) has reported 8 instances of untoward effects in young children, most of them with cyanosis. Of the 8, 2 had received suppositories. The other 6 received mixtures of drugs, one of which was acetophenetidin.

Soehring and Tautz (454) have reviewed the literature on the harmful effects of acetophenetidin and concluded that the condition was very easy to detect and that the incidence was much less frequent than after some other analgesic drugs. Most are agreed that the margin of safety is great. Moeschlin (337) observed a woman who recovered after she took at one time 200 tablets of a mixture containing a total of 50 g. acetophenetidin.

N-Acetyl-p-aminophenol. Batterman and Grossman (251) observed that untoward reactions were insignificant in a study of a large series of patients given 0.3 to 0.6 g. of *N*-acetyl-*p*-aminophenol for 1 to 25 weeks. The results were comparable to those occurring after placebos.

Recently it has been reported by Spalton (460) that "More than two million doses of *N*-acetyl-*p*-aminophenol have already been given to humans, and there have been no authenticated reports of toxic effects." Colgan and Mintz (79) observed no side-effects from the administration of doses of 120 mg. *N*-acetyl-*p*-aminophenol four times a day for 2 weeks to children 1 to 4 years old.

Fatalities after Acetophenetidin Ingestion

There are some early reports in which death is said to have occurred in patients receiving large doses of acetophenetidin. Frequently however the report is not clear that this drug played a major role in the outcome. Many of the cases of toxic symptoms resulting from the ingestion of large doses of acetophenetidin for long periods of time have been described earlier under the effects on organ systems.

Page (365) discussed a fatal case from a "current medical journal" but gave no reference. He named the reporter as a Dr. Tyler. The patient was a 32-year-old Italian, well-developed, suffering from an exanthema, who received 3.3 g. of acetophenetidin in 5 days. He also was given quinine sulfate, morphine, and Dovers powder. Certainly an adult with "measles" and who for clinical reasons was given so many potent drugs can scarcely be said to have died from this small amount of acetophenetidin.

Krönig (256) described a 17-year-old printer's apprentice who had complained of pain in the back of the head. He had been very pale in color, presumably due to lead poisoning from his work. The patient took four 1-g. doses of acetophenetidin in a 3 week period. On taking the fifth dose he had severe vomiting, became extremely weak, had blue-gray coloration of the lips and face, temperature 39°C., weak pulse, headache, and diarrhea. The liver and spleen were enlarged and easily palpable. The abdomen was extremely sensitive to deep palpation. There was a severe infection in the right external ear, and the ear drum was perforated. The body of the patient became increasingly yellow the following day while cyanosis was observed on the lips, ears, hands, and feet. The patient had a considerable increase in leucocytes and hemolysis in various stages with the red cells containing varying amounts of hemoglobin. The day after admission he died. The physician assumed that the patient had been weakened by sepsis and therefore had serious toxic effects from acetophenetidin which he normally tolerated well. Many of the symptoms and clinical findings suggest basic biliary tract disease. Krönig does not seem to have considered this. It will be recalled that the patient was not known to have ingested more than 4 g. of acetophenetidin in 3 weeks. During the discussion that followed the preceding one, Fraenkel (136) mentioned the case of a 17-year-old actress who received 1 g. of acetophenetidin and died that night. Further details were not given. White (515) discussed a case of acute dysentery in which death occurred from acute cardiac dilation, yet the physician associated the condition with chronic acetophenetidin poisoning. The man, 30 years old, was being treated for malaria. He had been given a 2.0-g. dose of ipecac with routine mustard leaf and tincture of opium. Vomiting occurred following this medication. There was blood and mucous in the stools, and the patient suffered abdominal cramps. Six days later, because of his heart condition, digitalis was started. The patient expired 3 days later. The patient was in the habit of taking 1 or more 0.3-g. tablets of acetophenetidin daily. However, none were found in his possession at the time of the death, and it was known that he had taken none for 10 days before his illness. Some evidence was presented to show that he had taken 200 g. of the drug in less than 60 days. The author stated that the patient died of acute dysentery, but that failure of a dilated heart was the ultimate cause of death. He also expressed the opinion that the severe depression and the rapid dilation could be fairly attributed to the use of acetophenetidin. The case record does not support this opinion.

Russow (407) discussed what he believed to be a death from acetophenetidin in a woman who had been perfectly normal and healthy until she complained of pain in her whole body after lightning had struck near her. A diagnosis of muscle rheumatism was made and the patient was given 1 g. of acetophenetidin twice daily along with 0.2 g. caffeine sodium benzoate. That evening she was pale, with profuse sweating and vomiting, exhibiting intense pain. After being given morphine, she was quieter but she still complained of the pain. Since she became steadily worse she was admitted to the clinic. She became unconscious, developed intense cyanosis of the face and extremities and died late that evening. Apparently no thought was given to the history of lightning shock and its effects on the patient.

Tobey (481) reports the case of a 16.5-year-old girl with a headache and cold who took two headache tablets, found later to contain acetophenetidin. An hour and 40 min. later she began to turn blue, and the physician found her with a weak heart and edema of the lungs. She died immediately. Of the 7 fatal cases reported in 1909 by Kebler *et al.* (238) in their survey of the harmful effects of various drugs, including acetophenetidin, one was that of a patient with pneumonia who received 4.7 g. daily for 2 days and who died suddenly. Another patient with influenza had received 0.3 g. every 3 hours but not over 6 doses. Still another was a patient with bronchitis of 1 year's duration who received 0.13 g. every 3 hours for 5 doses and who died 12 hours after the last dose; while a patient with typhoid fever died after receiving 0.17 g. every 2 hours until 8 doses had been taken. There were two cases in which acetophenetidin was given for headache. The first patient succumbed after taking 0.7 g.; the second one, who had a cerebral tumor, died after two 0.3-g. doses had been given 2 hours apart.

Cohen (78) reviewed cases of intoxication attributed to acetophenetidin. He concluded there had been only 7 cases due to overdosage reported in the American literature since 1892. He discussed the report by Kebler *et al.* and concluded that 6 of these cases had involved overdosage, 6 allergy, 8 idiosyncrasy, and 3 intoxication. He concluded that in 18 other cases there had been no evidence of intoxication.

Costen (85) reported the case of a 64-year-old woman who suffered from a fractured femur, who regularly took large doses of aspirin, acetophenetidin, and bromide. She developed scanning speech, tremor, and other signs of Parkinson's disease. She appeared to be convalescing without incident until she exhibited a daily temperature elevation and complained of malaise. Five days later there appeared a swelling about the right tonsil with a small lemon-yellow patch of exudate on its surface. Hematological studies showed a leucocyte count of 1840 per mm.^{3} with 50 per cent granulocytes, leading to a diagnosis of agranulocytic angina. She was irradiated over the long bones after removal of the cast. The temperature subsided, the blood counts rapidly became normal, and the pharynx became free of inflammation. She was discharged from the hospital with a white count of 9600 per mm.^{3} with 70 per cent granular cells. For 1 month she was free of symptoms with the leucocyte counts within normal limits and then she was readmitted to the hospital with a white count of 2600 per mm.^{3}, a temperature of 39.4°C., and a sloughing necrosis with gangrene of the pharynx. Daily irradiation of the long bones was given again but with no apparent response. The leucocyte count dropped to 200 and the patient expired. The physician believed that the regular ingestion of drugs for long periods was evidence in itself that this habit of hers was the chief factor in depressing bone marrow function. No mention was made of the possible role of irradiation in the disorder, nor did he specify the drugs employed together with the quantity and duration of their use. Holst (213) reported the case of a patient diagnosed as suffering from acetophenetidin intoxication, but the cause of death presumably was cancer of the colon.

Lowy (291) compiled the reports of the habitual use of barbiturates and analgesic drugs which were furnished by various hospitals throughout the United States. Out of 2.5 million admissions per year over a 10-year period, there were 16 cases attributed to acetophenetidin intoxication, among which 3 deaths were said to have occurred. These figures are compared with 117 cases recorded as acetanilid intoxication with 12 deaths and 74 cases wherein aspirin intoxication was suggested and among which 4 deaths were reported.

In a case reported to be due to chronic acetophenetidin ingestion, Espersen (120), at autopsy, found evidence of bronchopneumonia, cirrhosis of the liver, and ascites. Sears (429) observed a patient who took as much as 8 to 12 g. of aspirin, 5 to 8 g. of acetophenetidin, and 1.0 to 1.7 g. of caffeine per day over a 6-year period. Upon physical examination he had prominent ascites, moderate anemia, no cyanosis, tabes, and heart findings consistent with heart block with a frequency of 30. Later he developed a tachycardia, and an infusion of digitalis was given; the pulse rate fell to 80 in 36 hours, and he was clinically improved, but he died suddenly without struggle. At autopsy the right ventricle was found to be greatly distended with an organized thrombus in the right auricular appendage. The left ventricular wall was thickened; the coronary arteries were nearly obliterated but with no thrombi. The aorta displayed atherosclerosis which extended from arch to bifurcation and on into the femoral arteries. Renal findings indicated vascular disease. Death was believed to be due to extensive vascular degeneration with sudden reappearance of heart block. This patient was known to have had a luetic condition. The pathological findings were not traced to the overuse of drugs.

In 1957 there was a report by Allies (5) of death in a 10-day-old infant who had ingested a mixture of not more than 0.08 g. acetophenetidin, 0.08 g. acetylsalicylic acid, and 0.003 g. codeine. At autopsy there was evidence of hemorrhage in the kidneys and gastrointestinal tract. No history of the patient is given so there is no clue to the need for medication and no description of the clinical findings prior to administration of the drug. There is no mention of methemoglobinemia, a condition usually associated with the ingestion of toxic amounts of the drug.

No consistent pathological changes have been observed in the human after the administration of acetophenetidin. Most patients have some complaint for which they take the drug. Large doses of acetophenetidin may produce cyanosis but no grave pathological changes have been established as having been caused by the drug.

Therapy of Toxic Effects

No one has made a detailed study of the therapy of overdoses of acetophenetidin since the need has never been established. Meurice

(327,328) treated a patient simply by hot applications to extremities and along the limbs, and by administration of 1 g. of caffeine and 5 g. of sodium bicarbonate during the day. With this treatment the symptoms observed in his patient improved slightly, and the cyanosis receded. The author was not able to conclude whether the addition of sodium bicarbonate was helpful. In one case of reported poisoning (391), glucose solution was injected but this did not reverse the methemoglobinemia as had been reported by Brooks and Moldenhauer. Lesser (272) suggests that in acute poisoning the stomach pump and other supportive measures might be used. Jasinski and Müller (231) believed that ascorbic acid was effective in stopping the cyanosis. They also used iron salts which they believed resulted in an increase in hemoglobin. In one case which presented a low hemoglobin (471), the patient responded promptly to iron therapy. Wuhrmann and Jasinski (525), believing that an iron deficiency was associated with acetophenetidin intoxication, suggested that patients who had a hypochromic anemia also should be treated with vitamin B_{12}. This raises the question as to whether the diagnosis should not have been "hypochromic anemia" in a patient who has been taking acetophenetidin because of the clinical findings observed. All available evidence in the literature indicates that recovery from overdosage is rapid after discontinuance of the drug.

Acute Toxicity in Animals

Earthworms. Sollmann (456) found that a 1:50,000 solution of acetophenetidin was fatal to earthworms whereas they did survive a concentration of 1:75,000. Acetanilid was fatal in a 1:5000 solution, as was aspirin. The author concluded that earthworms were not reliable test objects of the clinical toxicity of antipyretics.

Frogs. Specker (461) gave frogs, weight not specified, 50 mg. of the drug. There was no effect in 2 hours but 3 days later they were dead.

Chickens. Éloy (117) gave a hen 2.0 g. of the drug per kg. and observed no toxic phenomena.

Mice. Hesse (198) gave the drug orally to mice with the following results: a dose of 1300 mg. per kg. produced no deaths in 11 animals; with 1500 mg. per kg., 3 of 6 died in 2 days; and with 1750 mg. per kg., 2 of 8 died in 2 days. Pohle and Spieckermann (381) stated the lethal dose of the drug to be 25 mg. per 20-g. mouse.

Pohle and Vogel (382) and Pohle and Dittrich (380) cited this same figure but none of these three papers contained any original data. Hesse *et al.* (199) found that the acutely toxic dose orally was 1.5 g. per kg. Brownlee and Gaddum (54) gave the drug orally to male and female mice fasted for 24 hours and weighing 18 to 24 g. The average lethal dose was calculated to be 1.38 g. per kg., compared with 1.36 g. per kg. for aspirin, and 3.23 g. per kg. for acetanilid. The LD_{50} of acetophenetidin in mice was found to be 2400 mg. per kg. (142). Ogiu *et al.* (357) found that the intraperitoneal LD_{50} of acetophenetidin was 650 mg. per kg., and Feeney *et al.* (127) found it to be 760 mg. per kg. Berger (28) found the LD_{50} of acetophenetidin to be 820 mg. per kg. with an LD_1 of 295 mg. per kg. Another report (333) gives the LD_{50} by intraperitoneal injection in mice as 902 mg. per kg.

Stegagno (466) studied the antagonism of barbiturates and acetophenetidin in mice. His results, with doses as high as 200 mg. of sodium *N*-methyl-cyclohexenyl-methyl-barbiturate per kg. and 1900 mg. of acetophenetidin per kg., did not demonstrate antagonism.

Rats. Gilman and Barbour (155) gave the drug to rats orally in an acacia suspension 18 hours after the removal of food. A dose of 4.0 g. per kg. produced 8 deaths among 15 animals during a 48-hour observation period, and 6.0 g. per kg. killed all in a group of 8 in the same time interval. Brownlee and Gaddum (54) gave the drug orally to young adult, male and female rats, weighing 150 to 200 g., after a 24-hour fast. The average lethal dose was calculated to be 820 mg. per kg. for acetanilid and 1250 mg. per kg. for acetophenetidin. Hart (189) gave the drug orally in a suspension in gum tragacanth and approximated the LD_{50} graphically. The LD_{50} of acetophenetidin in rats was 2.6 g. per kg. while that of acetanilid was 1.7 g. per kg., that of aspirin was 1.5 g. per kg., and that of salicylamide was 1.4 g. per kg. Eagle and Carlson (108) gave acetophenetidin to a group of albino rats, 75 per cent of them males, weighing 120 to 200 g. The drug was given orally in a suspension of 2 per cent acacia after an 18-hour fast. The rats were fed at the end of the experimental day and observed for 1 week thereafter. Using 111 rats the LD_{50} was found to be 1705 mg. per kg. whereas that of aspirin was 1360 mg. per kg. Renault *et al.* (393) found the LD_{50} to be 3.5 g. per kg.

Guinea pigs. Käer and Loewe (234) observed that in a mixture of barbital and acetophenetidin, the two components appeared to be antagonistic in their toxic actions but synergistic in their depressant effects. Loewe (287) found that in a mixture, acetophenetidin and codeine were antagonistic in their mutual toxicity. Also Loewe *et al.* (288) observed that the ingredients in a mixture of acetophenetidin, aspirin, and codeine detoxified each other to a certain extent. Hesse *et al.* (202) gave guinea pigs a dose of 800 mg. of acetophenetidin per kg. and observed no toxicity. A dose of 1000 mg. per kg. also produced no effect in 4 animals, but when he gave the same dose to 5 others one of them died within a period of 5 days.

Rabbits. Mahnert (307) found that death occurred after 16 hours when he gave 3 g. of the drug to a 1-kg. rabbit. Another rabbit weighing 650 g. was given 4.5 g. of the drug and died after 30 hours. Garcia y Mansilla (147) gave a rabbit weighing 860 g., 1.5 g. of acetophenetidin by stomach tube and, although he observed some effects, it is not recorded that the animal died. He gave another rabbit weighing 1010 g. an emulsion of 3.0 g. of the drug by stomach tube, and the animal died 6 hours later, while a third animal weighing 650 g. died 8 hours after 4.0 g. of the drug had been given. Rosen (403) observed that 1 g. of acetophenetidin killed a healthy rabbit in 1 hour and 16 min. Warren and Werner (506) stated that a dose of 800 mg. of acetophenetidin per kg. was fatal in 1 of 6 rabbits.

Dogs. In early work, Cerna and Carter (70) gave 5.0 g. of acetophenetidin to a 28-kg. dog and observed a gradual fall in blood pressure until death. They observed a similar response in a 5.8-kg. dog given 1 g. of acetophenetidin intravenously. The lethal dose was estimated to be 0.26 g. per kg. Hinsberg and Treupel (207) gave a dog weighing 5.3 kg., 2.4 g. of acetophenetidin corresponding to 0.45 g. per kg. body weight. By the following day the animal was normal in appearance. Free *et al.* (138) gave a dog 1 g. of acetophenetidin per kg. orally and observed that death occurred after about 10 hours.

A summary of the acute toxic doses in animals is given in Table 6.

N-Acetyl-p-Aminophenol

Frogs. Hinsberg and Treupel (207) gave a Hungarian frog weighing 100 g., 50 mg. of *N*-acetyl-*p*-aminophenol subcutaneously and found it dead the next morning. Another frog which was given 100 mg. per kg. died in 25 min.

TABLE 6
Acute Toxic Doses of Acetophenetidin in Various Species of Animals

Animal	Route of administration	LD_{50} mg. per kg.	Fatal dose mg. per kg.	Ref.
Frogs			50 (per frog)	(461)
Mice	Oral	1500 or more		(198)
Mice		1250		(381)
Mice	Oral		1500	(199)
Mice	Oral	1380		(54)
Mice		2400		(142)
Mice	Intraperitoneal	650		(357)
Mice	Intraperitoneal	820		(28)
Mice	Intraperitoneal	902		(332)
Mice	Intraperitoneal	760		(127)
Rats	Oral	4000		(155)
Rats	Oral	1250		(54)
Rats	Oral	2600		(189)
Rats	Oral	1705		(108)
Rats		3500		(393)
Guinea pigs	Oral	>1000		(202)
Rabbits		> 800		(506)
Rabbits		Aprox. 3000		(393)
Dogs	Intravenous		260	(70)

Mice. The LD_{50} of *N*-acetyl-*p*-aminophenol in mice was found to be 610 mg. per kg. (142). The LD_{50} of *N*-acetyl-*p*-aminophenol, when given orally to mice, was found to be 717 mg. per kg. (334).

Rats. Greenberg and Lester (162) gave large doses of *N*-acetyl-*p*-aminophenol orally to albino rats and observed that, with a dose of 4.0 g. per kg., death resulted within 24 hours. Various values have been given for the LD_{50} of this drug. Clark (74) found the LD_{50} of *N*-acetyl-*p*-aminophenol to be greater than 3200 mg. per kg. Free *et al.* (138) found that the oral LD_{50} in rats was about 3000 mg. per kg. It has, however, also been reported to be 1944 mg. per kg. (334) and 4500 mg. per kg. (393).

Guinea pigs. Hinsberg and Treupel (207) gave a guinea pig weighing 461 g., 1.5 g. of *N*-acetyl-*p*-aminophenol orally, and it was dead after 12 hours.

Rabbits. A female rabbit weighing 1950 g. received a total of 7.0 g. of *N*-acetyl-*p*-aminophenol intravenously in small doses. After 3.0 g. had been given there was a slight convulsion and after 4 hours and 10 minutes, and 7.0 g. of the drug, there was respiratory arrest

(207). Renault *et al.* (393) found the LD_{50} to be about 3.0 g. per kg.

Dogs. Hinsberg and Treupel (207) gave a dog 0.5 to 1.0 g. per kg. of the drug without fatal effect.

A summary of the acute toxic doses in animals is given in Table 7.

TABLE 7
Acute Toxic Doses of *N*-Acetyl-*p*-Aminophenol in Various Species of Animals

Animal	Route of administration	LD_{50} mg. per kg.	Fatal dose, mg. per kg.	Ref.
Frogs	Subcutaneous		100–500	(207)
Mice		610		(142)
Mice	Oral	717		(334)
Rats	Oral		4000	(162)
Rats		>3200		(74)
Rats	Oral	3000		(138)
Rats	Oral	1944		(334)
Rats		4500		(393)
Guinea pigs	Oral		3250 or less	(207)
Rabbits	Intravenous		3600 or less	(207)
Rabbits		Approx. 3000		(393)

The acute fatal dose in animals varies appreciably with the species and the manner of administration. Not surprisingly, the dose is higher when it is given orally rather than intraperitoneally. The fatal dose of *N*-acetyl-*p*-aminophenol in experimental animals is similar to that of acetophenetidin.

Chronic Toxicity

Mice. Aronson (15) found that acetophenetidin, in a concentration of 2 per cent in the diet, was lethal to mice in a few days.

Rats. Boughton and Stoland (41) gave acetophenetidin daily in therapeutic doses throughout the life cycle of albino rats. Drug feeding was started at the age of 10 weeks, and from this time until the animals were 200 days old, they were given 4.3 mg. per kg. daily. This dose was doubled when the animals were from 200 to 300 days of age. From 300 days to the end of the experimental period they received 12.9 mg. per kg. All the drugs tested were fed in milk. Acetophenetidin and acetanilid were given to male animals only, six in the group, for a total feeding period of 86 weeks. Acetophenetidin and acetanilid did not produce any observable effects during the first

72 weeks. At about the 72nd week both groups began to show evidence of toxicity. The appetites of the animals decreased rapidly, and they began to lose weight. They became hunched and dejected in appearance, and paid little attention to their care. The control groups remained normal in every respect. Although drug feeding was stopped at the beginning of the 76th week, there was no correction of symptoms during a 5-week abstinence interval. Both test groups were losing ground rapidly when the experiment was terminated. The authors believed that this was evidence that the toxic effects were permanent. A type of rat pneumonia, however, caused a number of deaths during the experiment. Three of the 6 animals getting acetophenetidin died of this as did 25 per cent of the control group.

Dogs. Espinosa (121) injected subcutaneously a dog weighing 2.5 kg. with 1.0 g. of acetophenetidin the first day, the second day with 0.25 g., and the third day with 0.5 g. The fourth day the author gave an intravenous dose of 2.5 g., and within a few minutes the dog had clonic convulsions followed by tonic convulsions. He reported that 2 more dogs were subjected to the same treatment with the same results. Masetti (318) gave a small, young dog weighing 5 to 6 kg. acetophenetidin by mouth. In the first experiment he gave 50 mg. per day to the animal and gradually increased the dose until he was giving 5.0 g. per day. Death came 15 days after he started the drug. In the second experiment he intended to kill the animal and started by giving 1.5 g. of acetophenetidin per day for 6 days. On the seventh or eighth day he increased the dose to 8.0 g. a day. The animal died on the morning of the ninth day. The total amount of acetophenetidin given was 13 g. In another experiment he started giving a dog 0.6 g. per day and increased the dose by 0.5 g. every 10 days. In $2^1/_2$ months he had reached a daily dose of 3.5 g. Since the animal was in a very poor state of health by this time, he discontinued the drug entirely. Ten days later the animal had completely recovered.

Human. Symptoms and pathological findings in the human due to the long continued ingestion of acetophenetidin are given under the effects on organ systems.

In experimental animals given large doses of the drug over long periods of time most of the pathological effects have been those associated with alterations of the blood and its pigments. No other effects have been demonstrated experimentally, even with doses far in excess of those ordinarily used in the human.

Chapter XI

Tolerance and Habituation

Since acetophenetidin was soon recognized to be relatively nontoxic, and since it has been available to the laity for a long time for self-medication, it is reasonable to expect that a patient who did not get relief from pain with small doses, or perhaps who experienced increasing pain with the extension of the pathological process, would take more and more of the drug. This in itself can hardly be termed tolerance.

The literature does not contain evidence that, under any circumstances, patients required greater doses or more frequent medication to secure relief for any stated condition. Mahnert (308) in discussing the early use of the drug, recommended giving one large dose at the height of the fever and a second at the start of a recurrence, since with small doses he got tolerance. This may have been due to the fact that the small doses were not sufficient to bring about antipyresis. Müller (345–348), who tried to produce a permanently lowered temperature by repeated doses, said that as much as 8 g. per day were not effective because tolerance developed. Burkhalter (58) observed that tolerance developed occasionally but was able to avoid it by stopping the acetophenetidin and administering another drug. After this, readministration of acetophenetidin produced better results.

Clark (73) discussed some of the early clinical reports in which the question of tolerance had been raised in relation to the analgesic and antipyretic drugs, including acetophenetidin. In some cases patients were said to have taken progressively larger doses, usually, however, for the relief of persistent pain. Goodman and Gilman (160) conclude that "tolerance to the analgesic action of acetanilid and acetophenetidin probably does not occur in man, but this point is disputed."

Undoubtedly a number of patients, many of them with recurring pain, such as headaches, become accustomed to taking something to relieve their discomfort. There is no evidence that the use of analgesic drugs for "headache" or other functional pain or for that matter when taken for temporary relief of pain from organic lesions has led to the physical and psychological dependence upon the drug which is characteristic of addiction.

Davis (92) discussed 3 cases of addiction to what he described as coal-tar derivatives. A woman had been taking acetophenetidin regularly for several months for relief of headache. She lost her supply accidentally and by the next day was in a hysterical condition, pale, with convulsive attacks and vomiting. Her respiration was rapid and spasmodic, and she was covered with cold perspiration. Her pupils were enormously dilated. It is not recorded whether these clinical findings were similar to those previously exhibited by the patient during a severe headache. The physician gave her 50 mg. of morphine sulfate, 1.2 mg. of atropine and digitalin. This quieted her for about 15 min., but it was necessary to repeat the morphine in an hour. After this she slept several hours, and a supply of acetophenetidin was obtained for her. Another patient had been taking about 1.0 to 1.3 g. daily for 7 months. Although anemic she refused to discontinue the drug. Kebler *et al.* (238) reported that he believed several of the analgesic drugs, including acetophenetidin, to be habit forming, but he did not present scientific evidence in support of his opinion. Dressen (100) mentioned that a mixture containing codeine phosphate, 0.01 g., aspirin, 0.25 g., acetophenetidin, 0.25 g., and nux col. pulv., 0.05 g., was well absorbed and effective, and did not produce habituation. Fisher (131) discussed chronic acetanilid poisoning and reported a case of a 47-year-old man who had taken large amounts of acetanilid and acetophenetidin. He had been taking the acetanilid for more than 20 years. Upon admission to the hospital the patient was extremely weak, cyanotic, with constant headache, tremors, and a marked tendency to sleep. He was confused, anorexic, and constipated. One week after the drugs had been discontinued he became confused and irrational, developing ideas of reference and persecution. The mental symptoms gradually disappeared in the course of the next week or two. Two months after withdrawal of the drugs he had gained 15 pounds, and his tremors and headaches had disappeared. It was stated that the patient had been confused upon admission to the hospital but that this condition was not adequately distinguished from those mental symptoms which he still showed even after he was no longer taking the acetophenetidin and acetanilid.

Clark (73) pointed out that almost all the evidence in favor of habituation to acetophenetidin and other analgesic drugs came from clinical reports, the majority of which were descriptions of cases in which the drugs were taken for pain that persisted or recurred after discontinuation of the drug.

According to Goodman and Gilman, "addiction apparently does not occur" and "physical dependence and withdrawal symptoms have not been demonstrated in animals and man. Reported clinical cases of addiction leave much to be desired in the way of convincing evidence."

In answer to the question, "Is acetophenetidin habit forming," the following reply is given in the *Journal of the American Medical Association* (13): "The answer depends on one's concept of 'drug habit' and 'withdrawal symptoms.' There are infinite gradations between the 'habit' of chewing gum, at one extreme, and heroin addiction at the other. 'Withdrawal symptoms' similarly grade insensibly from mild desire and discomfort to intense craving and physical collapse. Most people take acetophenetidin, acetanilid, or acetylsalicylic acid only occasionally and for definite indications such as headache, pain, or colds. Those who have habitual headache are inclined to take drugs habitually and may develop chronic poisoning, especially cyanosis, but they can stop without marked craving or other withdrawal symptoms. A few individuals appear to feel positive elation or even inebriation and these are more likely to use the drugs to excess and to feel the withdrawal more keenly and may object quite vigorously, especially if they have a neurotic or hysterical temperament, but violent reactions are rare and may be charged to inherent nervous irritability more than to these drugs."

Chapter XII

Summary

History

Acetophenetidin was introduced as an antipyretic drug in 1887. The salicylates had been in use only a few years, and acetanilid was introduced just one year earlier. This was at a time when it was generally believed that fevers in themselves were harmful and the use of antipyretic drugs was common. Within a year after acetophenetidin was introduced, there were reports from many countries of beneficial effects from its use as an antipyretic. As with many important drugs introduced during the last century or earlier, acetophenetidin was in common use before there were controlled pharmacological and clinical studies. The early clinical reports stressed its effectiveness and lack of undesirable side-effects. This led to its common use in large doses. It was not uncommon to find that patients were receiving 4 to 6 g. of the drug a day.

The use of *N*-acetyl-*p*-aminophenol is of much more recent date and followed the demonstration that it was the major metabolite of acetophenetidin and of acetanilid.

Metabolic Fate of Acetophenetidin

It was not until 1949 that adequate methods were devised for determining acetophenetidin and its metabolic products in biological fluids. The observations and experiments on the distribution and fate of the drug prior to this time should be interpreted with caution since they were not based on present-day methods of evaluation. With the use of these methods it was demonstrated that acetophenetidin was completely absorbed from the gastrointestinal tract. The highest levels of acetophenetidin occur about 2 hours after administration and little remains in the body after 5 hours. After absorption it is metabolized rapidly. One hour after administration to the human most of the acetophenetidin has been converted to *N*-acetyl-*p*-aminophenol and some of this already has been conjugated, presumably with glucuronic acid. The acetyl group stays on the molecule so that either in man or in experimental animals little more than 0.1 per cent of the compound is changed to *p*-phenetidin. A fraction of the acetophenetidin in the plasma is bound to the plasma proteins; at low concentrations this may be more than 50 per cent of the total concentration.

When *N*-acetyl-*p*-aminophenol is given orally it is rapidly absorbed, the rate of absorption being increased by the simultaneous administration of sodium citrate. Maximal plasma levels may be obtained as soon as 30 min. after oral administration and these decrease slowly, significant amounts being present 8 hours after administration. In experimental animals the concentrations of *N*-acetyl-*p*-aminophenol in the brain and in the plasma are approximately equal, even within 30 min. after oral administration. This suggests both rapid absorption and diffusion or secretion into the cerebro spinal fluid and is evidence that the drug reaches the central nervous system within a very short time after oral administration.

Antipyretic Action

Acetophenetidin rapidly found a place in therapy as an antipyretic drug and was accepted quickly as worthy of a place among the standard remedies of its time. When it first became available it was tried in many different kinds of fever, a number of them associated with infectious diseases. It was soon realized that the drug was effective against the fever but had no demonstrable action against the underlying infection. The drug reduced the fever no matter from what cause and was usually free from side-effects. In patients without fever it produced no effect on body temperature. It did not cause nausea, vomiting, or depression of the appetite, nor did it have adverse effects on the circulation. In high therapeutic doses it did not produce cyanosis or collapse.

The antipyretic action of acetophenetidin and *N*-acetyl-*p*-aminophenol has been easy to demonstrate in experimental animals. Many mixtures containing acetophenetidin or *N*-acetyl-*p*-aminophenol have been found to be effective as antipyretics, and there is some evidence that the antifebrile activity is markedly enhanced by including in the mixture one of the barbiturates.

Analgesic Action

Although introduced as an antipyretic drug, it quickly became apparent that acetophenetidin was effective in relieving the pain of migraine, sciatica, neuralgia, and rheumatoid arthritis. Despite many attempts to devise adequate methods for studying analgesia in experimental animals and in the human, it has been difficult to evaluate the action. No procedure in animals or in the human has gained wide acceptance. Experimental methods that have been employed in the human include electrical stimulation of the skin or of the tooth pulp and heat stimulation by focusing the light from a strong lamp onto the blackened forehead of normal subjects. The acknowledged clinical effectiveness of the drug in the relief of pain and the failure to demonstrate this by the experimental reduction of induced pain has led some to suggest that the drug may counteract pathological processes, which produce pain secondarily, both in headache and in arthritis. In this respect, the results that have been obtained in studies on acetophenetidin do not differ from those obtained with other nonnarcotic analgesic drugs such as the salicylates. Few drugs enjoy such wide use as analgesics, both in the clinic and in the home. It is a matter of common knowledge that acetophenetidin is effective in headache, and generalized aches and pains of muscle and joint origin.

A large number of substances have been given in combination with acetophenetidin for use as analgesic drugs. Common mixtures include acetophenetidin, aspirin and caffeine and acetophenetidin, aspirin, caffeine and codeine, but almost all of the other common nonnarcotic analgesic drugs and the barbiturates have been used in combination with acetophenetidin.

The experimental evidence for the effectiveness of *N*-acetyl-*p*-aminophenol as an analgesic is smaller in quantity but there is no reason to believe that it is not as effective as acetophenetidin.

Other Therapeutic Uses

Acetophenetidin has been used for a number of other conditions including rheumatoid arthritis, in which, in addition to its antipyretic effects, it causes a decrease in the swelling of the joints. Mixtures with one of the barbiturates have commonly been prescribed as hypnotics and sedatives. Aside from its use as an analgesic in upper respiratory infections, certain experimental studies suggest that it diminishes the duration of illness in influenza. In experimental animals it prolongs the hypnotic action of barbital.

Numerous experimental studies have failed to demonstrate the effectiveness of acetophenetidin against experimental tuberculosis, against spontaneous or transplanted tumors, or against the poliomyelitis virus.

Effects on the Central Nervous System

In the human there is little evidence that the drug has any significant central effects such as hypnosis, euphoria, loss of hearing, or elevation of convulsive threshold. Even in large doses it has no tendency to produce nausea or vomiting. Symptoms of tinnitus or vertigo are rare and ordinarily do not occur even after relatively large doses. There is less evidence concerning the effects of *N*-acetyl-*p*-aminophenol, but the data available do not indicate any significant central depressant effects.

Effects on the Cardiovascular System

In spite of the use of very large doses of the drug when it first became available, there were few reports that it had a depressant effect upon the heart. In some cases, when used in patients with a high fever, the temperature was reduced to far below the normal level and this, with the concomitant reduction in pulse rate, sometimes was misinterpreted as cardiac depression. The evidence suggests that neither acetophenetidin nor *N*-acetyl-*p*-aminophenol, even in relatively large doses, has an appreciable effect upon the heart or blood pressure unless given intravenously in high concentrations.

Effect on Erythrocytes

Many of the older reports in the literature concerning anemia are difficult to assess because the patients were ill with various diseases and had taken a number of different drugs. In more recent reports most of the patients have been women, and the authors have suggested that many of them were suffering from an iron deficiency.

There has been renewed interest in the possibility that large doses of acetophenetidin given for a long time may produce a moderate anemia. A significant contribution to this problem has been the demonstration that significant hemolytic anemias may occur in an occasional individual and these sensitive subjects may be detected on the basis of the capacity of their red cells to form specific inclusion bodies under the influence of certain drugs. These sensitive individuals suffer from a specific enzyme abnormality. There is general agreement that the bone marrow is not depressed and rapid and complete recovery from the anemia occurs as soon as the drug is withdrawn.

Cyanosis frequently is mentioned in the earlier literature in patients that have received large doses of acetophenetidin. Sometimes this has been due to altered blood pigments after the long-continued use of the drug, and at other times it can be attributed to the low body temperature produced by the very large doses of the drug in fever patients. Both in the early and recent reports cyanosis was associated with the ingestion of large doses of the drug and not with the ingestion of moderate doses. It is well to remember that cyanosis refers merely to a blue appearance which, in itself, is not an adequate sign of drug intoxication and, indeed, may be unrelated to its principal pharmacological and toxicological action.

In the early clinical reports, when large doses of acetophenetidin were used, there was an inadequate demonstration of the presence of methemoglobin and it was not well differentiated from other pigments. It occurs rarely in individuals taking moderate doses of drug, even for a long period of time. When normal subjects were given large doses of the drug the maximal concentration of methemoglobin was 2 to 3 per cent of the total hemoglobin. Even this small quantity disappeared gradually as the concentration of acetophenetidin in the plasma decreased. When medical students were given large doses of *N*-acetyl-*p*-aminophenol, the maximal methemoglobin concentration was only about $^1/_3$ of this or approximately 1 per cent.

Sulfhemoglobin is a poorly defined blood pigment which does not occur in normal blood, and apparently there is no mechanism for converting it to hemoglobin as there is in the case of methemoglobin. From the beginning it has been obvious that large doses of acetophenetidin for a long period of time are required to produce significant amounts of sulfhemoglobin. Any sulfhemoglobin formed disappears more slowly than methemoglobin. It appears probable that *N*-acetyl-*p*-aminophenol, even in large doses, is less apt to produce sulfhemoglobin.

Effects on Leucocytes

There are no well documented reports of the diminution of white cells after the administration of either acetophenetidin or *N*-acetyl-*p*-aminophenol. It may be concluded that there is no evidence of the depression of bone marrow activity after the administration of therapeutic doses of either drug and neither one has been demonstrated to produce a complete absence of white cells. Earlier reports associating diminished leucocyte counts with the administration of drugs sometimes mentioned acetophenetidin along with the others, but there is no evidence, even when patients are given large doses of the drug for a long period of time, that there is a significant depression of the leucocyte count. Such reports as there are of the occurrence of low leucocyte counts following the administration of acetophenetidin or *N*-acetyl-*p*-aminophenol do not seem to have excluded the effect of other factors. Certainly there is no demonstrated relationship between the ingestion of the drug and the leucocyte count.

Effects on Respiration

Neither in the human nor in experimental animals is there evidence that moderate doses of acetophenetidin or *N*-acetyl-*p*-aminophenol produce any significant effects upon the respiratory system.

Effects on Renal Function

It was appreciated very early that acetophenetidin had no effects on renal function. In some cases where patients have received large doses of the drug, along with several others, over a long period of time, there are reports claiming renal damage, but it is not evident that acetophenetidin was the causative agent.

Effects on Liver

Even when there have been clinical signs of acetophenetidin intoxication, such as cyanosis and anemia, the size of the liver and spleen have been found to be normal. Experimental studies in animals reveal no effects upon liver function.

Effect on Enzyme Systems

Most of the studies in isolated systems have revealed no effect of acetophenetidin on enzyme systems. This has been particularly significant in studies on the enzyme systems responsible for oxidative phosphorylation since salicylates act as uncoupling agents in this system but acetophenetidin does not.

Toxicology

It is not surprising that, with the widespread use of acetophenetidin, and in the early days in very large doses, there have been occasional untoward effects reported. Often, however, it has been very difficult to separate the effects of the acetophenetidin from those of other drugs given concurrently and to separate the toxic effects of the drugs from those associated with the disease in which the drugs were being used. Although skin disorders have been reported in patients given acetophenetidin, in most of the patients the evidence is not convincing that the drug was implicated.

There are some earlier reports in which death is said to have occurred in patients receiving large doses of acetophenetidin. Frequently, however, the report is not clear that acetophenetidin played a major role in the outcome. In this regard it is well to remember the caution (193) that "the incrimination of certain drugs has been by inference and on the basis of association rather than on the basis of absolute proof."

In experimental animals given large doses of the drug over long periods of time most of the pathological effects have been those associated with alterations of the blood and its pigments. No other effects have been demonstrated experimentally, even with doses far in excess of those ordinarily used in the human. Large doses of acetophenetidin may produce some methemoglobin in the human but no other pathological changes have been established as having been caused by the drug. No one has made a detailed study of the therapy of overdoses of acetophenetidin since the need has never been established.

Habituation

The majority of clinical reports of habituation to acetophenetidin are descriptions of cases in which the drug was taken for pain that persisted or recurred after discontinuation of the drug. There is no evidence that addiction occurs and physical dependence and withdrawal symptoms have not been demonstrated either in animals or in man.

Bibliography

1. Adams, W. L., R. Morrissey, D. Baker, and B. B. Clark, The effects of repeated doses of acetanilid and of acetophenetidin on dogs, *J. Pharmacol. Exptl. Therap.*, *69*, 274 (1940).
2. Ainlay, G. W., Palliative treatment of dysmenorrhea with acetylsalicylic acid, phenacetin and propadrine hydrochloride, *Am. J. Obstet. Gynecol.*, *39*, 83–86 (1940).
3. Albrecht, H., Klinische Erfahrungen mit Dolviran–Kinder und Säuglingszäpfchen, *Medizinische*, *1955*, 225–26.
4. Albricht, I. C., Über eine experimentelle quantitative Untersuchung der schmerzstillenden Wirkung verschiedener Analgetica, *Acta Brevia Neerl. Physiol. Pharmacol. Microbiol.*, 9, 109–10 (1939).
5. Allies, F., Iatrogene Phenazetinintoxikation bei Säuglingen, *Med. Klin. (Munich)*, *52*, 50–51 (1957).
6. Anonymous, Studies in therapeutics. VI. Paraphenacetin, *Brit. Med. J.*, *1888*, *I*, 1126.
7. Anonymous, The value of phenacetin, *Univ. Med. Mag.*, *1*, 182 (1889).
8. Anonymous, Phenacetin in typhoid fever, *Lancet*, *1890*, *2*, 31.
9. Anonymous, Pharmacology and therapeutics: adulteration of phenacetin, *Lancet*, *1890*, *2*, 1347.
10. Anonymous, Unpleasant effects of phenacetin, *Clinic of the Month*, 444 (1893).
11. Anonymous, Phenacetin (acetophenetidin) vs. acetanilid, *J. Am. Med. Assoc.*, *47*, 1923–24 (1906).
12. Anonymous, Current comment, Acetanilid, *J. Am. Med. Assoc.*, *87*, 103 (1926).
13. Anonymous, Is acetophenetidin habit forming? *J. Am. Med. Assoc.*, *115*, 798 (1940).
14. Archer, H. E. and G. Discombe, Sulphaemoglobinaemia. Its cause and prevention, with special reference to treatment with sulphanilamide, *Lancet*, *1937*, *2*, 432–35.
15. Aronson, H., Ueber die Wirkungsweise saurer Antifebrin und Phenacetinderivate, *Deut. med. Wochschr.*, *47*, 1285–86 (1891).
16. Averbuck, S. H., Über die Diuresehemmung durch Antipyretika, *Arch. exptl. Pathol. Pharmakol.*, *157*, 335–41 (1930).
17. Axelrod, J., The enzymic cleavage of aromatic ethers, *Biochem. J.*, *63*, 634–39 (1956).
18. Ayers, T. W., Therapeutic value of phenacetine, *Med. Record*, *35*, 541–42 (1889).
19. Ayers, T. W., Therapeutic value of phenacetine, *Trans. Med. Assoc. Alabama*, 319–24 (1890).
20. Baccarani, U., Ricerche comparative sull'eliminazione della urea, dell'-

acido solforico combinato e sulla tossicita urinaria, in seguito alla somministrazione della criofina e fenacetina, *Riforma med.*, *3*, 411–12 (1899).
21. Baer, M., Ueber Veronazetin, ein aus mehreren Komponenten zusammengesetztes Hypnotikum und Sedativum, *Münch. med. Wochschr.*, *59*, 472–73 (1912).
22. Baldi, D., Azione fisiologica della fenacetina, *Terap. mod. (Roma)*, *4*, 25–32 (1890).
23. Barthelmes, H., Dolviran in der kinderärztlichen Praxis, *Med. Klin. (Munich)*, *50*, 786–87 (1955).
24. Bateman, A. G., and 21 others, editors. Acetophenetidin, *Medical Annual and Practitioners Index*, 6th year, John Wright and Co., Bristol; and Hamilton Adams and Co., London, 1888, xvi, 619 pp.
25. Batterman, R. C., and A. J. Grossman, Analgesic effectiveness and safety of *N*-acetyl-*para*-aminophenol, *Federation Proc.*, *14*, 316–17 (1955).
26. Beecher, H. K., The measurement of pain, *Pharmacol. Rev.*, *9*, 59–209 (1957).
27. Bell, R., Phenacetine, *Brit. Med. J.*, *1888*, *I*, 744.
28. Berger, F. M., Hypnotic action resulting from combined administration of salicylamide and acetophenetidin, *Proc. Soc. Exptl. Biol. Med.*, *87*, 449–51 (1954).
29. Bergstermann, H., A. Kerschensteiner, and J. Schmidt., Untersuchungen der analgetischen und spasmolytischen Eigenschaften des Hyodon, *Münch. med. Wochschr.*, *95*, 122–23 (1953).
30. Bernheim, F., *The interaction of drugs and cell catalysts*, Burgess Publishing Co., Minneapolis, 1942, iii, 85 pp.
31. Bertran, E. C., and F. S. Sanchez, Modificaciones farmacologicas de la fosfomonoesterasa acida hepatica canina, *Arch. inst. farmacol. exptl. (Madrid)*, *3*, 110–16 (1951).
32. Betts, W. A., A case of phenacetin idiosyncrasy, *Brit. Med. J.*, *1896*, *I*, 146.
33. Beutler, E., R. J. Dern, and A. S. Alving, The hemolytic effect of primaquine. VI. An *in vitro* test for sensitivity of erythrocytes to primaquine, *J. Lab. Clin. Med.*, *45*, 40–50 (1955).
34. Biernacki, J., The general management and special treatment of the commoner fevers, *Med. Times and Hosp. Gaz.*, *25*, 557–58 (1897).
35. Blumenthal, L. S., M. Fuchs, and A. Bennett, Headache clinic. V. Tension headache, *Am. Practitioner and Dig. Treatment*, *4*, 701–06 (1953).
36. Boone, U. S., Antipyrine, acetanilide and phenacetin. Are they harmful remedies? Are they habit-forming drugs? Thesis, St. Louis, Missouri, 1910, ii, 44 pp.
37. Boréus, L.-O., and F. Sandberg, The analgesic and antipyretic action of the combination of acetophenetidin and barbital, *Acta Physiol. Scand.*, *28*, 6–13 (1953).
38. Boréus, L.-O., and F. Sandberg, A comparison of some pharmacological effects of acetophenetidin and *N*-acetyl-*p*-aminophenol, *Acta Physiol. Scand.*, *28*, 261–66 (1953).
39. Boréus, L.-O., and F. Sandberg, The analgesic action of *N*-acetyl-*p*-amino-

phenol and of its combination with some other substances, *Acta Physiol. Scand.*, *28*, 266–71 (1953).

40. Boréus, L.-O., F. Sandberg, and E. Agren, Experimental and clinical studies on the synergism and antagonism of oral analgesics, *Acta Odontol. Scand.*, *13*, 219–34 (1956).
41. Boughton, L. L., and O. O. Stoland, The effects of drugs administered daily in therapeutic doses throughout the life cycle of albino rats, *Univ. Kansas Sci. Bull.*, *27*, 27–60 (1941).
42. Boutaric, A., and J. A. Gauthier, Action inhibitrice des composés antithermiques sur quelques réactions d'oxydation, *J. pharm. chim.*, *27*, 97–105 (1938).
43. Boyd, L. J., W. Gittinger, and J. Schwimmer, Sleep induction with combined administration of salicylamide and acetophenetidin, *N. Y. State J. Med.*, *57*, 924–28 (1957).
44. Brandenburg, R. O., and H. L. Smith, Sulfhemoglobinemia: A study of 62 clinical cases, *Am. Heart J.*, *42*, 582–88 (1951).
45. Brodie, B. B., and J. Axelrod, The physiological disposition of acetophenetidin (*p*-ethoxyacetanilide) in man, *Federation Proc.*, *7*, 207–08 (1948).
46. Brodie, B. B., and J. Axelrod, The estimation of acetanilide and its metabolic products, aniline, *N*-acetyl-*p*-aminophenol and *p*-aminophenol (free and total conjugated) in biological fluids and tissues, *J. Pharmacol. Exptl. Therap.*, *94*, 22–28 (1948).
47. Brodie, B. B., and J. Axelrod, The fate of acetanilide in man, *J. Pharmacol. Exptl. Therap.*, *94*, 29–38 (1948).
48. Brodie, B. B., and J. Axelrod, Metabolic fate of acetophenetidin in man, *J. Pharmacol. Exptl. Therap.*, *97*, 58–67 (1949).
49. Brodie, B. B., J. Axelrod, J. R. Cooper, L. Gaudette, B. N. La Du, C. Mitoma, and S. Udenfriend, Detoxication of drugs and other foreign compounds by live microsomes, *Science*, *121*, 603–04 (1955).
50. Brody, T. M., Action of sodium salicylate and related compounds on tissue metabolism *in vitro*, *J. Pharmacol. Exptl. Therap.*, *117*, 39–51 (1956).
51. Brown, E. A., Drug allergy, *Quart. Rev. Allergy and Appl. Immunol.*, *7*, 51–82 (1953).
52. Brownlee, G., A comparison of the antipyretic activity and toxicity of phenacetin and aspirin, *Quart. J. Pharm. and Pharmacol.*, *10*, 609–20 (1937).
53. Brownlee, G., The role of the aromatic amino group in deranged pigment metabolism, *Biochem. J.*, *33*, 697–708 (1939).
54. Brownlee, G., and J. H. Gaddum, A therapeutic index for the coal-tar antipyretics with an appendix on the accuracy of a cross-over test, *Quart. J. Pharm. and Pharmacol.*, *12*, 45–65 (1939).
55. Bruns, F., F. Hahn, and W. Schild, Untersuchung zur Pharmakologie der Waermeregulation, I. Ueber den Wirkungsmechanismus und die Angriffspunkte der Narkotika, Krampfgifte unde Antipyretika, *Arch. exptl. Pathol. Pharmakol.*, *209*, 104–29 (1950).
56. Brunton, T. L., *Lectures on the action of medicines. Being the course of*

lectures on pharmacology and therapeutics, Macmillan Co., New York, 1899, xv, 673 pp.
57. Burge, W. E., The effect of pyretics and antipyretics on catalase production, *J. Pharmacol. Exptl. Therap., 14,* 121–30 (1919).
58. Burkhalter, E., *Phenacetin als Antipyreticum,* Inaugural Dissertation, Basel, 1889, 64 pp.
59. Burrill, D. Y., F. R. Goetzl, and A. C. Ivy, The pain threshold raising effects of amphetamine, *J. Dental Research, 23,* 337–44 (1944).
60. Busch, E., Erfahrungen mit Eu-Med, *Med. Klin. (Munich), 26,* 1299 (1930).
61. Cachin, M., F. Pergola, and F. Pottet, Intoxication aiguë par la phenacétine avec methémoglobinémie, *Bull., soc. méd. hôp. Paris, 72,* 693–95 (1956).
62. Caldwell, W. C., Antipyretics, *North Am. Practitioner, 4,* 225–32 (1892).
63. Carló, P. E., N. M. Cambosos, G. C. Feeney, and P. K. Smith, Plasma levels after the oral administration of acetylsalicylic acid and *N*-acetyl-*p*-aminophenol in different forms to human subjects, *J. Am. Pharm. Assoc., Sci. Ed., 40,* 396–99 (1955).
64. Carslaw, J. H., Phenacetine as an antipyretic, *Glasgow Med. J., 30,* 64–67 (1888).
65. Carson, P. E., C. L. Flanagan, C. E. Ickes, and A. S. Alving, Enzymatic deficiency in primaquine-sensitive erythrocytes, *Science, 124,* 484–85 (1956).
66. Carter, F. W., An unusual case of poisoning, with some notes on non-alkaloidal organic substances, *Med. J. Australia, 1936, II,* 558–64.
67. Cass, L. J., W. S. Frederick, and J. B. Andosca, A clinical evaluation of a new buffered analgesic agent, *Am. J. Gastroenterol., 26,* 576–81 (1956).
68. Cattani, C., La Fenacetina, *Gazz. med. ital., 1,* 365–69; 375–78; 385–86; 398–99; 408–11; 415–18; 425–27; 435–37; 445–49; 465–68; 475–78 (1888).
69. Cerna, D., Phenacetin as a toxic agent, *J. Am. Med. Assoc., 24,* 711–12 (1895).
70. Cerna, D., and W. S. Carter, A study of the comparative actions of antipyrine, phenacetine and phenocoll on the circulation and heat phenomena, *Notes on New Remedies, 5,* 49–67 (1892).
71. Cerny, M., Über Gefahren der Phenacetinmedikation im Säuglingsalter, *Praxis, 29,* 634–37 (1950).
72. Cesari and Burani, Sur l'acétophénétidine ou phénacétine, *Bull. gén. thérap.,* 525–26 (1888).
73. Clark, B. B., Symposium: Can the euphoria, analgetic and physical dependence effects of drugs be separated? III. The non-opiate analgesics, *Federation Proc., 2,* 195–201 (1943).
74. Clark, B. B., *N*-acetyl-*p*-aminophenol. A, Pharmacological studies. B, Cardiovascular and metabolic studies in laboratory animals and man, *Symposium on N-acetyl-p-aminophenol, The Institute for the Study of Analgesic and Sedative Drugs,* Elkhart, Ind., 1952, pp. 23–37.
75. Cleaves, R. L., Antipyretics in continued fevers, *Trans. Iowa State Med. Soc., 10,* 84–89 (1892).

76. Clemmesen, C., Forgiftning efter overdosering med "blanede hovedpine-pulvere," *Ugeskrift Laeger, 95,* 766 (1933).
77. Čmuchal, J., On the action of phenacetin, *Casopis lékáru českých., 28,* 191–94; 214–17; 233–36 (1899).
78. Cohen, A., *Acetophenetidin,* Philadelphia, 1940, pamphlet, 36 pp.
79. Colgan, M. T., and A. A. Mintz, The comparative antipyretic effect of *N*-acetyl-*p*-aminophenol and acetylsalicylic acid, *J. Pediat., 50,* 552–55 (1957).
80. Collischonn, Phenacetin als Antirheumaticum, *Deut. med. Wochschr., 16,* 97–98 (1890).
81. Collischonn, Zur Wirkung der Thyangol-Pastille, *Med. Klin. (Munich), 24,* 1990–91 (1928).
82. Conklin, R. L., Summary of clinical use of *N*-acetyl-*p*-aminophenol, *Symposium on N-acetyl-p-aminophenol, The Institute for the Study of Analgesic and Sedative Drugs,* Elkhart, Ind., 1952, pp. 66–67.
83. Conkling, H., Discussion of West, F. E., Note on the therapeutics of certain modern antipyretics, *Brooklyn Med. J., 7,* 352–65 (1893).
84. Cornely, D. A., and J. A. Ritter, *N*-acetyl-*p*-aminophenol (Tylenol elixir) as a pediatric antipyretic-analgesic, *J. Am. Med. Assoc., 160,* 1219–21 (1956).
85. Costen, J. B., Agranulocytosis: appearance of the early pharyngeal lesion; three cases, one apparent recovery, *Ann. Otol. Rhinol. and Laryngol., 42,* 372–84 (1933).
86. Coxon, R. V., and J. P. Crawford, Sulphaemoglobinaemia following prolonged administration of phenacetin, *Brit. Med. J., 1940, II,* 556.
87. Cramer, J. S. N., Dampfdruckbestimmungen an einigen organischen Stoffen, *Rec. trav. chim., 62,* 606–10 (1943).
88. Crohn, W. H., Ein schwerer Fall von Ueberempfindlichkeit, *Med. Klin. (Munich), 26,* 1451 (1930).
89. Crombie, A., Notes on the comparative value of antipyrin, antifebrin and phenacetin as antipyretics, *Indian Med. Gaz., 24,* 193–200 (1889).
90. Cronk, G. A., D. E. Naumann, K. McDermott, P. Menter, and M. B. Swift, A controlled study of the effect of oral penicillin G in the treatment of non-specific upper respiratory infections, *Am. J. Med., 16,* 804–909 (1954).
91. Davies, D., Clinical testing of analgesics, *Acta Pharmacol. Toxicol., 10,* 113–16 (1954).
92. Davis, J. S., A report of three cases of addiction to coal tar derivatives, *Am. Medico-Surg. Bull., 7,* 1490–1493 (1894).
93. Davison, C., J. Stern, B. J. Britt, and P. K. Smith, Comparative studies on aspirin and *N*-acetyl-*p*-aminophenol, unpublished observations, 1956.
94. Demme, Ueber die Wirkung und Dosirung der hauptsächlichsten neueren Antipyretica, mit Beziehung auf das Kindesalter, *Therap. Monatsh. Berlin, 5,* 160 (1891).
95. Dennig, A., Ueber die Einwirkung einiger vielgebrauchter Arzneimittel auf die Methämoglobinbildung im Blute, *Deut. Arch. klin. Med., 65,* 524–41 (1900).
96. Dern, R. J., E. Beutler, C. L. Flanagan, and A. S. Alving, Studies of the

acute hemolytic anemia induced by certain aniline derivatives and related compounds, *J. Lab. Clin. Med., 44,* 788 (1954).

97. Dern, R. J., E. Beutler, and A. S. Alving, The hemolytic effect of primaquine. V. Primaquine sensitivity as a manifestation of a multiple drug sensitivity, *J. Lab. Clin. Med., 45,* 30–39 (1955).
98. DeSanctis, R. W., C. Williams, G. O. Barnett, and C. DuToit, The medical grand rounds Massachusetts General Hospital Case 344, Sulfhemoglobinemia, *Am. Practitioner and Dig. Treatment, 7,* 807–10 (1956).
99. Dreser, H., Die Bestimmung der respiratorischen Kapazität kleiner Blutmengen, *Arch. exptl. Pathol. Pharmakol., 61,* 138–49 (1908).
100. Dressen, M., Über meine Erfahrungen mit "Phenalgetin," *Med. Klin. (Munich), 25,* 1938–39 (1929).
101. Duca, C. J., R. D. Williams, and J. V. Scudi, Chemotherapy of tuberculosis. III. *In vitro* and *in vivo* activities of various compounds, *Proc. Soc. Exptl. Biol. Med., 67,* 159–62 (1948).
102. Dujardin-Beaumetz, M., Propriétés et indications de la phénacétine, *Bull. mém. soc. thérap., 15,* (2), 203–04 (1888).
103. Dujardin-Beaumetz, M., De l'acétophénétidine ou phénacétine, *Semaine méd., 8,* 132 (1888).
104. Dujardin-Beaumetz, M., Des phénacétines, *Semaine méd., 8,* 398–99 (1888).
105. Dujardin-Beaumetz, M., On the phenacetins. (Abstract paper read annual meeting Brit. Med. Assoc., Glasgow, Aug. 1888) *Post Graduate, 5,* 66–68 (1889).
106. Dujardin-Beaumetz, M., On the phenacetins (translation), *Brit. Med. J., 1889, I.,* 521–22.
107. DuToit, C. H., personal communication, 1956.
108. Eagle, E., and A. J. Carlson, Toxicity, antipyretic and analgesic studies on 39 compounds including aspirin, phenacetin and 27 derivatives of carbazole and tetracarbazole, *J. Pharmacol. Exptl. Therap., 99,* 450–57 (1950).
109. Ebbinghaus, H., Vergleichende Untersuchungen über die schmerzstillende Wirkung einiger Antipyretica, Inaugural Dissertation, Münster, 1934, 31 pp.
110. Eddy, N. B., Studies of morphine, codeine and their derivatives, *J. Pharmacol, Exptl. Therap., 45,* 339–59 (1932).
111. Editorial, La phénacétine, *Union méd.,* No. 152, pp. 889–93 (1891).
112. Editorial, The harmful effects of acetanilid, antipyrin, and phenacetin, *J. Am. Med. Assoc., 53,* 303 (1909).
113. Edlefsen, G., Zum Nachweise des Phenetidins im Harn, *Centr. inn. Med., 21,* 2–5 (1900).
114. Eisenhart, H., Leichte Phenacetinintoxication, *Therap. Monatsh., 7,* 252 (1893).
115. Eldridge, C. S., Phenacetine, *Times and Register, 30,* 205–07 (1895).
116. Eldridge, C. S., Various uses of phenacetine, *Med. Surg. Reporter, 74,* 300–03 (1896).
117. Éloy, Ch., Les propriétés et la valeur therapeutique des phénacétines, *Gaz. hebd. méd. chir.,* 39, 610–14 (1888).

118. Enders, A., W. Hertlein, and M. Wiedersheim, Die Wirkung von Phenacetin, Pyramidon, Coffein und Theobromin auf die normale und die durch Methylcellulose erhöhte Temperatur, *Arch. intern. pharmacodynamie, 94,* 416–25 (1953).

119. Ercoli, N., and M. N. Lewis, Studies on analgesics. I. The time-action curves of morphine, codeine, dilaudid and demerol by various methods of administration. II. Analgesic activity of acetylsalicylic acid and aminopyrine, *J. Pharmacol. Exptl. Therap., 84,* 301–17 (1945).

120. Espersen, T., Om den Chroniske phenacetin-forgiftning. Blodets udnytning ved phenacetin-cyanosen. Ventilering af spørgsmaalet lever cirrhose paa basis af langvarig intoxication med anilinderivater, *Ugeskrift Laeger, 99,* 993–99 (1937).

121. Espinosa, N. M., Fenacetina, Thesis, Mexico, 1890, iv, 24 pp.

122. Falcone, C., and C. Gioffredi, Sopra una speciale localizzazione delle lesioni del sistema nervoso centrale nell'avvelenamento sperimentale da fenacetina, *Giorn. intern. sci. med. Napoli, 21,* 961–64 (1899).

123. Falk, E., Ueber Nebenwirkungen und Intoxicationen bei der Anwendung neuerer Arneimittel, *Therap. Monatsh., 4,* 314–15 (1890).

124. Faraggi, De la phénacétine, *Gaz. méd. d'Orient,* p. 44 (1888).

125. Faulkner, A. S., Notes on phenacetin in the treatment of continuous and malarious fevers and on sulphonal as an hypnotic, *Indian Med. Gazz., 24,* 227–29 (1889).

126. Fedotova, V. A., and N. I. K. Khorsova, Clinical chronic phenacetin intoxication, *Klin. med. (U.S.S.R.), 30,* 88 (1952).

127. Feeney, G. C., P.-E. Carló, and P. K. Smith, Action of salicylates and related compounds on carbohydrate metabolism and on adrenal ascorbic acid and cholesterol concentrations, *J. Pharmacol. Exptl. Therap., 114,* 299–305 (1955).

128. Fernández de Ybarra, A. M., Un caso de envenenamiento con fenacetina—curacion, *Gac. méd. Catalana, 15,* 229–30 (1892).

129. Fernández de Ybarra, A. M., A case of poisoning with phenacetine, *Med. Record, 41,* 108 (1892).

130. Finch, C. A., Methemoglobinemia and sulfhemoglobinemia, *New Engl. J. Med., 239,* 470–78 (1948).

131. Fisher, L. C., Chronic acetanilid poisoning, *J. Am. Med. Assoc., 100,* 736–37 (1933).

132. Fleisch, A., and M. Dolivo, Auswertung der Analgetica im Tierversuch, *Helv. Physiol. et Pharmacol. Acta, 11,* 305–22 (1953).

133. Flinn, F. B., and B. B. Brodie, The effect on the pain threshold of *N*-acetyl *p*-aminophenol, a product derived in the body from acetanilide, *J. Pharmacol. Exptl. Therap., 94,* 76–77 (1948).

134. Flodmark, S., Senidorm ett nytt barbitursyrefritt kombinationshypnoticum för åldringar, *Svenska Läkartidn., 51,* 128–33 (1954).

135. Forschelen, J., Beiträge zur Kenntnis der Wirkung des Phenacetins, Inaugural Dissertation, Bonn, 1888, 24 pp.

136. Fraenkel, A., *Berlin klin. Wochschr., 32,* 1000 (1895).

137. Frazer, T. H., Antipyretics; their uses and limitations, *Trans. Med. Assoc. Alabama,* 278–87 (1899).

138. Free, A. H., H. M. Free, M. H. Pindell, and V. K. Pittard, Biochemical and pharmacological studies with acetyl *para*-aminophenol and related compounds, Miles-Ames Research Lab., *Rept. No. 5212,* 27 (June 1952).
139. Friedman, A. P., and H. H. Merritt, Treatment of headache, *J. Am. Med. Assoc., 160,* 1111–17 (1957).
140. Friedman, A. P., and T. J. C. von Storch, Studies on vascular headache, one thousand cases of migraine and tension headache, *Southern Med. J., 46,* 1127–32 (1953).
141. Friedman, A. P., T. J. C. von Storch, and H. H. Merritt, Migraine and tension headaches, a clinical study of two thousand cases, *Neurology, 4,* 773–88 (1954).
142. Frommel, E., P. Gold, D. Melkonian, C. Radougo, J. Delmonte, F. Valette, and M.-B. de Quay, Le *N*-acétyl *p*-aminophénol, comparaison de l'effet antithermique et analgésique de ce corps à celui de l'antipyrine, de la phénacétine, du pyramidon et de la quinine, *Praxis, 46,* 968–72 (1953).
143. Gad, I., E. Jacobsen, S. Madsen, and K. Schmith. Undersøgelser over methaemoglobindannelse efter fenacetin og acet-4-kloranilid, *Ugeskrift Laeger, 112,* 1405–11 (1950).
144. Gaiffe, Sur les phénacétines, *Bull. gén. thérap., Paris, 115,* 71–76 (1888).
145. Gaiffe, V. de P.-X.-H., Étude sur les phénacétines. Thèse pour le Doctorat en Médecine, Paris, 1888, 39 pp.
146. Garbelli, G., Sull'impiego di un nuovo analgesico in ostetricia e ginecologia, *Minerva ginecol., 7,* 315–17 (1955).
147. Garcia y Mansilla, S., Estudio terapéutico sobre la fenacetina, *Rev. Clin. Hospitales, 2,* 145–315 (1890).
148. Garrano, F., Due casi di emicrania idiopatica ribelle, curati con il salofine e la fenacetina, *Boll. clin. Milano, 15,* 457–60 (1898).
149. Gates, M. F., A comparison of antipyretics, *Med. Times, 19,* 229 (1889).
150. Geisler, F. K., The question of the action of phenacetin in fever cases, *Vrachenbol Delo, 10,* 785–87; 840–41; 858–60 (1889).
151. Georgievsky, I., Acetophenetidin—new antifebril drug (translated from Russian), *Vrachenbol Delo, 5,* 83–85 (1888).
152. Gibson, Q. H., Methaemoglobin and sulphaemoglobin, *Biochem. J., 57,* iii (1954).
153. Gibson, R. D., T. S. Miya, and L. D. Edwards, A biological method for the evaluation of the non-narcotic analgesics, *J. Am. Pharm. Assoc., Sci. Ed., 44,* 605–07 (1955).
154. Gilman, A., and H. G. Barbour, Effects of phenacetin and aspirin respectively upon action of phenobarbital, *Proc. Soc. Exptl. Biol. Med., 32,* 1634–36 (1935).
155. Gilman, A., and H. G. Barbour, Antipyretic action in rats of tolysin alone and in combination with phenacetin, *Proc. Soc. Exptl. Biol. Med., 33,* 627–30 (1936).
156. Godelbarrer, A., Ueber Aethylsulfon-*p*-phenetidin, *Arch. intern. Pharmacodynamie, 23,* 3–15 (1913).
157. Goetzl, F. R., The experimental evidence for analgesic properties of antipyretic drugs. A critical review of literature with report on additional experiments, *Permanente Foundation Med. Bull., 4,* 49–63 (1946).

158. Goetzl, F. R., D. Y. Burrill, and A. C. Ivy, A critical analysis of algesimetric methods with suggestions for a useful procedure, *Quart. Bull. Northwestern Univ. Med. School, 17,* 280–91 (1943).

159. Goldbach, H. I., and R. Opfer-Schaum, Schnellverfahren zum toxikologischen Nachweis einiger Analgetica und Sedativa, *Pharmazie, 7,* 379–80 (1949).

160. Goodman, L. S., and A. Gilman, *The pharmacological basis of therapeutics,* 2nd ed., Macmillan Co., New York, 1955, xiii, 1831 pp.

161. Greenberg, L. A., and D. Lester, The metabolic fate of acetanilid and other aniline derivatives. I. Major metabolites of acetanilid appearing in the urine, *J. Pharmacol. Exptl. Therap., 88,* 87–98 (1946).

162. Greenberg, L. A., and D. Lester, The metabolic fate of acetanilid and other aniline derivatives. III. The role of *p*-aminophenol in the production of methemoglobinemia after acetanilid, *J. Pharmacol. Exptl. Therap., 90,* 150–53 (1947).

163. Greenleaf, R. W., Poisoning from headache powders, *Boston Med. Surg. J., 139,* 370–71 (1898).

164. Gregg, E. C., Jr., Effect of non-opiate analgesics and other drugs on the vibratory threshold, *J. Pharmacol. Exptl. Therap., 106,* 1–13 (1952).

165. Grenfell, H. O., The treatment of pyrexia with phenacetin, *Practitioner, 40,* 344–50 (1888).

166. Griffi, F., Comportamento di alcuni componenti urinari e dell'assorbimento intestinale in seguito a somministrazioni di alcune sostanze antipiretiche, *Biochim. e terap. sper., 27,* 233–61 (1940).

167. Guleke, H., Taubheit in Folge von Phenacetinmissbrauch, Z. *prakt. Aerzte, 8,* 765–66 (1889).

168. Guttmann, P., Über acetphenetidin, *Deut. Med. Z., 9,* 675 (1888).

169. Haffner, F., Experimentelle Prüfung schmerzstillender Mittel, *Deut. med. Wochschr., 55,* 731–33 (1929).

170. Hajnal, J., *N*-acetyl-*para*-aminophenol as an analgesic, *Brit. Med. J., 1956, II,* 1430–31.

171. Hald, J., Undersøgelser over acet-4-kloranilid som forurening i fenacetin, *Dansk. Tidskr. Farm., 24,* 113–95 (1950).

172. Hale, W., and G. P. Grabfield, The effect of certain drugs upon faradic sensibility, *J. Pharmacol. Exptl. Therap., 19,* 262 (1922).

173. Hale, W., and G. P. Grabfield, The action of certain depressant drugs on the sensory threshold for faradic stimulation in human subjects and the effect of tobacco smoking on this action, *J. Pharmacol. Exptl. Therap., 21,* 77–84 (1923).

174. Haller, J. F., Report of three hundred and fourteen cases of influenza, *Boston Med. Surg. J., 122,* 151–52 (1890).

175. Hambourger, W. E., Comparison of the antipyretic action and toxicity of *d*-glucono-*para*-phenetidin and acetophenetidin, *Proc. Soc. Exptl. Biol. Med., 31,* 365–67 (1933).

176. Hamill, P., and T. G. M. Hine, A case of phenacetin poisoning; recovery, *Lancet, 1915, 1,* 490–91.

177. Hamilton, R. R., Production of codeine, *Lancet, 270,* 322)1956).

178. Hammarsten, G., and O. Nordenfelt, Ett fall av kronisk acetanilid- och fenacetinförgiftning, *Nord. Med.*, *1*, 773–75 (1939).
179. Hanes, C. B., Evaluation of a non-narcotic analgesic preparation in private general practice, *Am. Practitioner and Dig. Treatment*, *7*, 602–04 (1955).
180. Hanzlik, P. J., Health hazards in acetanilide-containing nostrums and mixtures, *J. Am. Dental Assoc.*, *27*, 1505–12; 1672–78; 1833–38 (1940).
181. Hardy, J. D., H. G. Wolff, and H. Goodell, *Pain sensations and reactions*, Williams and Wilkins, Baltimore, 1952, xv, 435 pp.
182. Hare, H. A., *Fever, its pathology and treatment by antipyretics*, Davis, Philadelphia, *2*, 114–26 (1891).
183. Harold, J., Unpleasant effects of phenacetin, *Practitioner*, *53*, 444 (1894).
184. Harris, R., and J. C. Bird, Clinical evaluation of a new buffered aspirin, phenacetin and caffeine analgesic, *Clinical Med.*, *3*, 39–41 (1956).
185. Harris, S. C., and N. E. Brandel, The tooth pulp as an algesimetry site, *J. Dental Research*, *29*, 68–72 (1950).
186. Harris, S. C., and R. C. Worley, Human "analgesic" action of *d*-amphetamine, amobarbital, acetylsalicylic acid and acetophenetidin, in combination, *Proc. Soc. Exptl. Biol. Med.*, *83*, 515–18 (1953).
187. Harris, S. C., and R. C. Worley, Evaluation of a new analgesic, *J. Appl. Physiol.*, *7*, 84–88 (1954).
188. Harrop, G. A., Jr., and R. L. Waterfield, Sulphaemoglobinemia, *J. Am. Med. Assoc.*, *95*, 647–50 (1930).
189. Hart, E. R., The toxicity and analgetic potency of salicylamide and certain of its derivatives as compared with established analgetic-antipyretic drugs, *J. Pharmacol. Exptl. Therap.*, *89*, 205–09 (1947).
190. Hasegawa, A. T., and C. C. Pfeiffer, Effect of some antipyretic drugs on the glycosuria of alloxan diabetic rats, *Federation Proc.*, *12*, 329–30 (1953).
191. Haxthausen, H., Fixt, erythematost og pigmenteret Exanthem efter Codyl (Phenacetin), *Nord. Med.*, *38*, 713 (1948).
192. Healy, J. C., Sulphaemoglobinemia, *J. Lab. Clin. Med.*, *18*, 348–54 (1933).
193. Heck, F. J., Adverse effects of drugs on blood and bone marrow, *Med. Clin. N. Am.*, *1956*, 1077–90.
194. Heimann, R., Phenacetin, ein Mittel gegen Keuchhusten? *Münch. med. Wochschr.*, *207* (1889).
195. Heinroth, H., Über die Wirkung verschiedener Arzneimittel auf die Schmerzempfindlichkeit der Zahnpulpa, *Arch. exptl. Pathol. Pharmakol.*, *116*, 245–60 (1926).
196. Henry, J. P., Phenacetin in influenza, *Brit. Med. J.*, *1891*, *I*, 1282.
197. Henschen, S. E., Om s.k. konträr verkan af febermedel, *Upsala Läkareflören. Förh.*, *24*, 263–76 (1888–89).
198. Hesse, E., Zur biologischen Wertbestimmung der Analgetika und ihrer Kombinationen, *Arch. exptl. Pathol. Pharmakol.*, *158*, 233–46 (1930).
199. Hesse, E., E. Baumgart, and H. Dickmann, Zur Wirkungssteigerung der Schlafmittel durch Analgetica, *Klin. Wochschr.*, *11*, 1665–68 (1932).
200. Hesse, E., and H. Kuegler, Die biologische Wertbestimmung der Analgetika und ihrer Kombinationen, *Schweiz. med. Wochschr.*, *62*, 324–25 (1932).

201. Hesse, E., and H. Reichelt, Zur Wertbestimmung der Analgetika und ihrer Kombinationen, *Arch. exptl. Pathol. Pharmakol., 169,* 453–58 (1933).
202. Hesse, E., G. Roesler, and F. Buhler, Zur biologischen Wertbestimmung der Analgetika und ihrer Kombinationen. II. Mitteilung. *Arch. exptl. Pathol. Pharmakol., 158,* 247–53 (1930).
203. Heubner, X. W., Studien über Methaemoglobinbildung, *Arch. Exptl. Pathol. Pharmacol., 72,* 241–81 (1913).
204. Heubner, W., and W. Silber, Studien über die Prufung antipyretischer Mittel nebst Vergleich eines optisch aktiven Antipyrinderivates mit seinem Razemat, *Arch. exptl. Pathol. Pharmakol., 169,* 530–36 (1933).
205. Heusner, Ueber Phenacetin, *Therap. Monatsh., 2,* 103–04 (1888).
206. Hinsberg, O., and A. Kast, Ueber die Wirkung des Acetphenetidins, *Centr. med. Wiss. Berlin, 25,* 145–48 (1887).
207. Hinsberg, O., and G. Treupel, Ueber die physiologische Wirkung des *p*-Amidophenols und einiger Derivate desselben, *Arch. exptl. Pathol. Pharmakol., 33,* 216–50 (1894).
208. Hirschfeld, M., Ein Fall von chronischer Phenacetin-Vergiftung, *Deut. med. Wochschr., 31,* 66 (1905).
209. Hirschfelder, L., Beitrag zur Wirkung des Phenacetins, *Deut. Arch. klin. Med., 44,* 434–36 (1888–89).
210. Hoffmann, F., Über die analgetische Potenz von Acetylsalicylsäure und Salicylamid, *Arzneimittel Wochschr., 8,* 698–701 (1953).
211. Holladay, W. M., Art. IV. Phenacetin, an antifebrile and antineuralgic, *Virginia Med. Monthly, 15,* 640–42 (1888–89).
212. Hollopeter, W. C., Phenacetine poisoning, *Med. News, 55,* 335 (1889).
213. Holst, J. E., Chronisk phenacetinforgiftning, *Ugeskrift Laeger, 96,* 845–47 (1934).
214. Holtzem, M. J., Über die Kombination *p*-Aminobenzoesauresalizyl (Artesan A 55) in der Therapie rheumatischer Krankheiten, *Münch. med. Wochschr., 98,* 1698–99 (1956).
215. Hoppe, H., Ueber die Wirkung des Phenacetin (*para*-Acetphenetidin), *Therap Monatsh., 2,* 160–68 (1888).
216. Horanyi, M., and J. Rév, Serious anemia following abuse of Karil, *Orvosi Hetilap, 95,* 1090–92 (1954).
217. Horigeshi, S., Effects of several febrifuges on the movements of intestinal canal and uterus of live rabbits (translated from Japanese), *J. Chosen Med. Assoc., 26,* 1179–91 (1936).
218. Horikawa, Y., Studies on thiaminase in human feces. On the effects of various medicines upon thiaminosis, *Vitamins (Japan),* 3, 114–18 (1951).
219. Horváth, Á., Observations on the effects of phenacetin (translated from Hungarian), *Orvosi Hetilap, 37,* 473–75 (1889).
220. Horváth, Á., Beiträge zur Wirkung des Phenacetin, *Pester Med. Chir. Presse, 25,* 1134 (1889).
221. Hottenstein, C. D., *Univ. Med. Mag., 1,* 259–60 (1889).
222. Houde, R. W., personal communication, 1956.
223. Huet, In welchen febrilen Krankheiten ist die Verabreichung von Antipyretic nothwendig? *Münch. med. Wochschr., 36,* 655 (1889).

224. Humphreys, B. F., The uses and abuses of the new antipyretics, *Practitioner, 43,* 190–201 (1889).
225. Illoway, H., Does phenacetin possess convulsivant properties? *Med. News, 63,* 240–41 (1893).
226. Ivens, W. H. J., and J. M. van Vollenhoven, Over de intraglobulaire Sulfhaemoglobinae, *Ned. Tijdschr. Geneesk., 69,* 447–52 (1925).
227. Jaksch, R. v., Ueber die neueren Antipyretica und ihre Verwendung am Krankenbette, *Wien. med. Presse., 29,* 41–47 (1888).
228. Jaksch, R. v., Ueber die neueren Antipyretica und ihre Wirkung am Krankenbette, *Therap. Monatsh., 2,* 188–89 (1888).
229. Jasinski, B., Ueber zwei Fälle von toxischer, hämolytischer Anämie nach Phenacetin resp. Sulfonamiden, *Schweiz. med. Wochschr., 78,* 681–84 (1948).
230. Jasinski, B., Weitere Erkenntnisse zur Pathogenese der toxisch-hämolytischen Anämie nach Phenacetin (Saridon), *Schweiz. med. Wochschr., 80,* 1113–14 (1950).
231. Jasinski, B., and D. Müller, Zur Pathogenese der toxisch-hämolytischen Anämien nach chronischem Phenacetinabusus, *Schweiz. med. Wochschr., 80,* 681–84 (1950).
232. Jenkins, G. L., and W. H. Hartung, *The chemistry of organic medicinal products,* 3rd ed., John Wiley and Sons, New York, 1949, ix + 745 pp.
233. Johnson, J. R., J. M. Sheldon, K. P. Mathews, and R. G. Lovell, A clinical study of phenacetin-caffeine in the treatment of hay fever, *J. Allergy, 23,* 365–69 (1952).
234. Käer, E., and S. Loewe, Über Kombinationswirkungen. IV. Mitteilung: Die Wirkungsvariationen im Gemisch Veronal–Phenazetin, *Arch. exptl. Pathol. Pharmakol., 116,* 140–46 (1926).
235. Kallner, S., The cyanosis developing during treatment with sulfanilamide preparations, *Acta Med. Scand., Suppl., 130,* 1–110 (1942).
236. Kartschewski, A. J., Zur Frage von der Wirkung des Phenacetins bei Abdominaltyphus, *St. Petersburg med. Wochschr., 25,* 24 (1890).
237. Kast and Bamberger, cited by Richelot *et al.,* ref. 394.
238. Kebler, L. F., F. P. Morgan, and P. Rupp, The harmful effects of acetanilid, antipyrin, and phenacetin. *U. S. Dept. Agric. Bur. Chem. Bull. 126,* 85 pp., Government Printing Office, Washington, 1909.
239. Kibbe, M. E., Ecchymotic spots and pruritus due to phenacetin, *Occidental Med. Times, 15,* 371–72 (1901).
240. Kiese, M., Zur Pathochemie des Blutfarbstoffs, *Deut. Arch. klin. Med., 195,* 442–45 (1949).
241. Killian, J. A., Prolonged administration of mixtures containing *N*-acetyl-*p*-aminophenol to human subjects under observation, *Symposium on N-acetyl p-aminophenol, The Institute for the Study of Analgesic and Sedative Drugs,* Elkhart, Ind., 1952, pp. 52–56.
242. Klein, R., and H. Kremer, Klinische Erfahrungen mit dem oralen Analgetikum Melabon, *Wien, med. Wochschr., 104,* 1004–05 (1954).
243. Klemperer, J., Intusabletten, *Med. Welt, 3,* 1191–92 (1929).
244. Knowles, F. E., Symptoms of poisoning from a probable overdose of phenacetine, *Med. Record, 46,* 564–65 (1894).

245. Kobler, G., Das Acetphenetidin als Antipyreticum, *Wien. med. Wochschr.*, *37*, 865–68 (1887).
246. Kobler, G., Das Acetphenetidin als Antipyreticum, *Wien. med. Wochschr.*, *37*, 899–904 (1887).
247. Kondo, A., Blood vessels as affected by various aromatic substances. A comparison of the constitution of the drugs and their action (translated from Japanese), *Kyoto Igaku Zassi*, *14*, 1243–93 (1917).
248. Kracke, R. R., The experimental production of agranulocytosis, *Am. J. Clin. Path.*, *2*, 11–30 (1932).
249. Kracke, R. R., Relation of drug therapy to neutropenic states, *J. Am. Med. Assoc.*, *111*, 1255–59 (1938).
250. Kracke, R. R., and F. P. Parker, The etiology of granulopenia (agranulocytosis) with particular reference to drugs containing the benzene ring, *Am. J. Clin. Path.*, *4*, 453–69 (1934).
251. Kracke, R. R., and F. P. Parker, The etiology of granulopenia (agranulocytosis) with particular reference to the drugs containing the benzene ring, *J. Lab. Clin. Med.*, *19*, 799–818 (1934).
252. Kracke, R. R., and F. P. Parker, The relationship of drug therapy to agranulocytosis, *J. Am. Med. Assoc.*, *105*, 960–66 (1935).
253. Kracke, R. R., and F. P. Parker, Relation of drugs to the leukopenic state, *J. Med. Assoc. Georgia*, *25*, 51–57 (1936).
254. Kramer, P. E., M. L. Robbins, and P. K. Smith, Phenolic compounds as chemotherapeutic agents against poliomyelitis virus in tissue culture, *J. Pharmacol. Exptl. Therap.*, *113*, 262–71 (1955).
255. Krantz, J. C., Jr., and C. J. Carr, *The pharmacologic principles of medical practice*, 4th ed., Williams and Wilkins Co., Baltimore, 1958, xi, 1313 pp.
256. Krönig, G., Phenacetin-Vergiftung mit tödtlichem Ausgang, *Berlin klin. Wochschr.*, *32*, 998–1000 (1895).
257. Krönig, G., Phenacetinvergiftung mit tödlichem Ausgang, *Verhandl. Ver. inn. Med. Berlin*, *15*, 216–25; 235–38 (1895–96).
258. Krönig, G., Blutbefunde in je einem Falle einer tödtlich verlaufenen Phenacetin- und Kali-chloricum-Vergiftung, *Verhandl. Congr. inn. Med. Wiesb.*, *14*, 549–50 (1896).
259. Kulkarnt, S. B., Dielectric constant and dipole moment of some drugs, Part 1, *J. Indian Chem. Soc.*, *26*, 207–10 (1949).
260. La Belle, A., and J. A. Tornaben, Effects of various analgesics on inflammatory edema resulting from silver nitrate injection, *Science*, *114*, 187–88 (1951).
261. Lachowicz, E., On the action of phenacetin Bayer (*para*-acetophenetidin), *Przeglad Lekarski*, *27*, 274–76 (1888).
262. Lackie, J. L., Note on phenacetin as causing dyspnea and orthopnoea, *Med. Press and Circ.*, *60*, 208–09 (1895).
263. Lagutin, M. V., The mechanism of the depressing action of phenacetin (translated from Russian), *Farmakol. i Toksikol.*, *5*, 7–11 (1942).
264. Laporte, M. G., Un cas d'intoxication par la phénacétine, *France Service Santé Militaire*, *55*, 38–42 (1910).

265. Laurence, S. M., Case of poisoning by phenacetin and antikamnia, *Brit. Med. J., 1904, I,* 545.
266. Lazarus, S., Sulphaemoglobinaemia due to aniline derivatives, *Brit. Med. J., 1945, II,* 565–66.
267. Ledoux, Récherches sur l'action physiologique de la phénacétine, *Rev. méd.* (*Paris*), *12,* 313–16 (1892).
268. Lee, M. H., The local use of phenacetin, *Memphis Med. Monthly, 12,* 481–85 (1892).
269. Leech, D. J., and W. Hunter, An inquiry regarding the importance of ill-effects following the use of antipyrin, antifebrin, and phenacetin conducted by the therapeutic committee of the British Medical Association. *Brit. Med. J., 1894, I,* 85–90.
270. Lendon, G., The use and abuse of drugs, *Med. J. Australia, 1953, II,* 472–74.
271. Lépine, R., Sur le traitement de la fièvre typhoide; la phénacétine, *Semaine méd., 7,* 503–04 (1887).
272. Lesser, M. A., Acetophenetidin, *Drug and Cosmetic Ind., 51,* 35–37, 49 (1942).
273. Lester, D., Formation of methemoglobin. I. Species differences with acetanilide and acetophenetidine, *J. Pharmacol. Exptl. Therap., 77,* 154–59 (1943).
274. Lester, D., Formation of methemoglobin. II. Repeated administration of acetanilide and acetophenetidine, *J. Pharmacol. Exptl. Therap., 77,* 160–64 (1943).
275. Lester, D., and L. A. Greenberg, The metabolic fate of acetanilid and other aniline derivatives. III. Major metabolites of acetanilid appearing in the blood, *J. Pharmacol. Exptl. Therap., 90,* 68–75 (1947).
276. Lewin, L., *Ueber die Nebenwirkung der Arzneimittel,* A. Hirschwald, Berlin, 1893, pp. 549–54.
277. Lewis, J. R., Comparative study of phenacetin, thymacetin and an isomer, 4-ethoxy-2-isopropyl-5-methylacetanilide, *Arch. intern. pharmacodynamie, 93,* 450–55 (1953).
278. Liaci, L., Influenza di alcune sostanze antipiretiche sull' assorbimento intestinale, su vari componenti urinari e su alcune costanti fisicochimiche del sangue, *Arch. ital. sci. farmacol., 8,* 213–41 (1939).
279. Lim, R. K. S., and M. H. Pindell, A comparison of the antipyretic action of aspirin, phenacetin, acetyl-*para*-aminophenol and APC tablets in dogs, *Miles-Ames Research Laboratory, Rept. No. 5214* (August 5, 1952).
280. Lim, R. K. S., and M. H. Pindell, A comparison of the antipyretic action of sodium acetylsalicylate and acetyl-*para*-aminophenol in dogs, *Miles-Ames Research Laboratory, Rept. No. 5215,* 2 pp., 2 fig. (August 11, 1952).
281. Linckint, F., Phenan als Antineuralgicum, Antipyreticum und als Mittel zur Bekämpfung des Röntgen- und Alkohol-Nikotin-Katers, *Med. Welt., Berlin, 8,* 1695 (1934).
282. Lindmann, Unangenehme, bedrohliche Nebenwirkungen des Phenacetin, *Therap. Monatsh., 2,* 307–08 (1888).

283. Lipschitz, W., Über den Wirkungsmechanismus von Blutgiften, *Ergeb. Physiol.*, *23*, 1–32 (1924).

284. Livierato, P. E., Azione della fenacetina (acetofenetidina) sul ricambio materiale dell'uomo sano, *Riv. clin. ital. medica* (*Milano*), *28*, 358–64 (1889).

285. Löbl, V., Aspirin and phenacetin poisoning, *Budapesti Orvosi Ujság*, *2*, 803–806 (1904).

286. Loebisch, W. F., *Die neueren Arzneimittel in ihrer Anwendung und Wirkung*, Urban und Schwarzenberg, Wien und Leipzig, 1895, viii, 416 pp.

287. Loewe, S., Antineuralgische "Mischpulver," *Deut. med. Wochschr.*, *54*, 559–61 (1927).

288. Loewe, S., E. Käer, and H. Muischenk, Über Kombinationswirkungen. VII. Mitteilung: Grundlagen der Prüfung von Drei-Pharmakamischungen. Anwendung auf Phenazetin-Azetylsalizylsäure-Codeinmischungen, *Arch. exptl. Pathol. Pharmakol.*, *120*, 25–40 (1927).

289. Long, F. A., Treatment of the pyrexias by chemical antipyretics, *Gaillard's Med. J.*, *72*, 804–07 (1900).

290. Lowenstein, Veronazetin gegen Seekrankheit, *Münch. med. Wochschr.*, *62*, 1206 (1914).

291. Lowy, O., A comparative study of the habitual use of barbiturates and coal-tar derivatives as furnished by reports from various hospitals throughout the United States, *Can. Med. Assoc. J.*, *31*, 638–41 (1934).

292. Lüdecke, T., Zur Therapie von rheumatischen, neuralgischen, und grippösen Erkrankungen in der Allgemeinpraxis, *Med. Monatsschr.*, *7*, 47–50 (1953).

293. Lundsteen, E., E. Meulrengracht, and A. Rischel, Kronisk acetanilidforgiftning som folge af vedvarende brug af "blandede hovedpinepulvere" eller lignende kompositioner, *Ugeskrift Laeger*, *99*, 155–62 (1937).

294. Lundsteen, E., E. Meulengracht, and A. Rischel, Chronic acetanilid poisoning as the result of continuous use of "Mixed Headache Powders" or similar compounds, *Acta Med. Scand.*, *96*, 462–80 (1938).

295. MacGillycuddy, N., Phenacetin, *Brit. Med. J.*, *1891*, *II*, 190.

296. Macht, D. I., and W. Bloom, Effect of some antipyretics on the behavior of rats in the circular maze, *J. Pharmacol. Exptl. Therap.*, *17*, 21–40 (1921).

297. Macht, D. I., J. Greenberg, and S. Isaacs, The effect of some antipyretics on the acuity of hearing, *J. Pharmacol. Exptl. Therap.*, *15*, 159–65 (1920).

298. Macht, D. I., J. P. Greenberg, and S. Isaacs, Concerning the influence of antipyretics on the acuity of hearing, *Proc. Soc. Exptl. Biol. Med.*, *17*, 22–23 (1919–20).

299. Macht, D. I., S. Isaacs, J. P. Greenberg, On the influence of some antipyretics on the neuro-muscular coordination test of "tapping," *Proc. Soc. Exptl. Biol. Med.*, *15*, 61–62 (1915).

300. Macht, D. I., S. Isaacs, and J. P. Greenberg, On the influence of some opiates and antipyretics on the field of vision, *Proc. Soc. Exptl. Biol. Med.* *15*, 46–48 (1917).

301. Macht, D. I., S. Isaacs, and J. Greenberg, Action of some antipyretic analgesics on psychological reaction time, *Psychobiology I*, 327–38 (1917).

302. Macht, D. I., and M. B. Macht, Quantitative studies on pain threshold after administration of various drugs, *J. Am. Pharm. Assoc., Sci. Ed., 29,* 193–99 (1940).

303. Macon, W. L., Jr., Citrus bioflavonoids in the treatment of the common cold, *Ind. Med. and Surg., 25,* 525–27 (1956).

304. Macy, R., Partition coefficients of fifty compounds between olive oil and water at 20°C., *J. Ind. Hyg. Toxicol., 30,* 140–43 (1948).

305. Madison, F. W., and T. L. Squier, Further observations on the relation of amidopyrine to acute primary granulocytopenia, *Trans. Am. Therap. Soc., 34,* 76–79 (1934).

306. Madison, F. W., and T. L. Squier, The etiology of primary granulocytopenia (agranulocytic angina), *J. Am. Med. Assoc., 102,* 755–59 (1934).

307. Mahnert, F., Ueber Phenacetin vom klinischen und physiolgischen Standpunkte, *Deut. med. Wochschr., 14,* 1027–30 (1888).

308. Mahnert, F., Ueber Phenacetin vom klinischen und physiologischen Standpunkte, *Deut. med. Wochschr., 14,* 1048–51 (1888).

309. Maier, C., A. Bühlmann, and M. Hotz, Die O_2-Dissoziationskurve bei Sulf- und Methämoglobinämien, *Z. ges. exptl. Med., 118,* 105–08 (1951).

310. Maloney, A. H., Further studies in dilaudid medication, *J. Natl. Med. Assoc., 32,* 212–14 (1940).

311. Mandala, O., Influenze di solubilità (Costituzione chimica e solubilità), *Gazz. chim. ital., 56,* 896–901 (1926).

312. Mandewirth, P., Über die Wirkung einiger Antipyretika auf die Sauerstoffzehrung, Inaugural Dissertation, Münster, 1933, 19 pp.

313. Manicke, P., and P. Grigel, Zur Darstellung der Acetylsalicylsäure, des Acetanilids und des *p*-Acetphenetidins, *Arch. Pharm., 264,* 322–24 (1926).

314. Markovics, J., Erfahrungen mit Gelonida antineuralgica bei gynäkologischen Erkrankungen, *Med. Klin. (Munich), 25,* 720 (1929).

315. Martin, E., and Blumentritt, Curavon als Sedativum und Analgetikum, *Med. Welt, 2,* 1276–77 (1928).

316. Martin, E. G., C. M. Grace, and J. H. McGuire, The influence of drugs on the human sensory threshold, *J. Pharmacol. Exptl. Therap., 6,* 527–32 (1915).

317. Martin, G. J., The effect of various agents on the excretion of uric acid and allantoin, *Exptl. Med. Surg., 6,* 24–27 (1948).

318. Masetti, E., Le alterazioni nervose nell'avvelenamento sperimentale per fenacetina, *Soc. ital. med. int. (Roma), 9,* 459–63 (1899).

319. Masius, M., Contribution à l'étude des propriétés thérapeutiques de la phénacétine, *Bull. acad. roy. méd. Belg., 2,* 815–37 (1888).

320. Mays, T. J., Some clinical observations on the effects of the latest febrifuge, acetophenetidine, *Med. News, 51,* 204 (1887).

321. McGuigan, R. A., Pressor and other effects of antipyretics on digitalis action, *Proc. Soc. Exptl. Biol. Med., 38,* 314–15 (1938).

322. McLane, R. A., Clinical evaluation of combined drug therapy in acute upper respiratory infections, *J. Med. Soc. New Jersey, 49,* 509–10 (1952).

323. McLane, R. A., and C. C. Heck, Combined drug therapy in acute upper respiratory infections, *J. Med. Soc. New Jersey, 51,* 407–10 (1954).

324. Mering, von, J., Beiträge zur Kenntniss der Antipyretica, *Therap. Monatsh.*, *7*, 577–87 (1893).
325. Merlevede, E., Misbruik van Phenacetine en vorming van methaemoglobine, *Belg. Tijdschr. Geneesk.*, *8*, 289–98 (1952).
326. Meulengracht, E., and E. Lundsteen, Die Cyanose und Anämie bei chronischer Acetanilid-Vergiftung, *Folia Haematol.*, *63*, 89–99 (1939).
327. Meurice, J., Contribution a l'étude de la toxicité de la phénacétine, *Ann. soc. roy. méd. Gand*, *85*, 198–206 (1905).
328. Meurice, J., Contribution à l'étude de la toxicité de la phénacétine, *Belg. méd.*, *12*, 339–43 (1905).
329. Michaelis, Über Acetphenetidin, *Deut. med. Z.*, *9*, 675 (1888).
330. Michel, H. O., F. Bernheim, and M. L. C. Bernheim, The hydrolysis of acetanilide by various tissues, *J. Pharmacol. Exptl. Therap.*, *61*, 321–27 (1937).
331. Michelson, M. J., Action of narcotics upon the activity of choline esterase. IV. Narcotic power of different narcotics as compared with their inhibiting action upon the activity of choline esterase (translated from Russian), *Fiziol. Zhur. S.S.S.R.*, *32*, 745–56 (1946).
332. Miles Laboratories, Inc., Weekly report, physiology section (Dec. 7, 1954).
333. Miles Laboratories, Inc., Toxicity of Alka-Seltzer and Apamide-Ves (Jan. 11, 1955).
334. Miles Laboratories, Inc., Weekly report, physiology (Jan. 18, 1955).
335. Misrachi, De la phénacétine, *Gaz. Méd. d'Orient*, p. 43 (1888).
336. Misrachi and Rifat, Contribution à l'étude clinique et thérapeutique de la phénacétine (*para*-acetphénétidine), *Bull. gén. thérap.*, *114*, 481–97 (1888).
337. Moeschlin, S., Phenacetinsucht und -schäden, *Schweiz. med. Wochschr.*, *87*, 123–28 (1957).
338. Mönkemöller, Veronacetin als Hypnotikum und Sedativum in der psychiatrischen Praxis, *Psychiat.-Neurol. Wochschr.*, *14*, 572–74 (1913).
339. Montero Rodríguez, A., Intoxicatión por antitérmicos, análogo a un síndrome de Waterhouse-Friedrichsen, *Acta pediát. españ.*, *12*, 841–45 (1954).
340. Morinaka, K. Über den Einfluss der verschiedenen Antipyretica auf die Verteilung des Stickstoffs im Harn, *Z. physiol. Chem.*, *129*, 111–29 (1923).
341. Mörner, K. A. H., Fenacetinets omsättningsproduckter i menniskans organism, *Hyg. Festband.*, *14*, 1–7 (1889).
342. Mörner, K. A. H., Stoffwechselproducte des Acetanilids im menschlichen Körper, *Z. physiol. Chem.*, *13*, 12–25 (1889).
343. Morse, H. N., Ueber eine neue Darstellungsmethode der Acetylamidophenole, *Ber. deut. chem. Ges.*, *11*, 232–33 (1878).
344. Muirhead, A. L., The pharmacology of antipyretics, *Am. J. Clin. Med.*, *13*, 35–8 (1906).
345. Müller, F. R., Ueber Acetphenetidin, *Berlin. Klin. Wochschr.*, *30*, 613 (1888).
346. Müller, F. R., Ueber Acetphenetidin, *Deut. med. Wochschr.*, *14*, 661–62 (1888).
347. Müller, F. R., Über Acetphenetidin, *Deut. med. Z.*, *pp.* 674–75 (1888).

348. Müller, F. R., Ueber Acetphenetidin, *Therap. Monatsh.*, *2*, 355–58 (1888).
349. Münchau, H., Ueber die Wirkung des Coffeinzusatzes in schmerzstillenden Arzneimischungen, Inaugural Dissertation, Münster, 1934, 28 pp.
350. Murray, L. M., An analysis of sixty cases of drug poisoning, *Arch. Pediat.*, *43*, 193–96 (1926).
351. Nesnera, E., A simple abortive treatment of influenza, *Practitioner, 124*, 231–34 (1930).
352. Newton, D. R. L., and Tanner, J. M., *N*-Acetyl-*para*-aminophenol as an analgesic: A controlled clinical trial using the method of sequential analysis, *Brit. Med. J.*, *1956*, 1096–99.
353. Nissim, A., De la phénacétine, *Gaz. méd. d'Orient*, p. 44 (1888).
354. Noach, E. L., M. A. C. DeDie, and E. Kuipers, The influence of phenacetin on adrenal activity, *Acta Physiol. Pharmacol. Neerl.*, *5*, 8–27 (1956).
355. Noorden, C. von, Über Diäthylbarbitursäurekompositionen, *Therap. Monatsh.*, *33*, 413–16 (1919).
356. Öffinger, Aus Wissenschaft und Praxis. Eine eigenthümliche Nebenwirkung des Phenacetin, *Ärztl. Mitt. Baden-Karlsruhe*, *43*, 110–11 (1889).
357. Ogiu, K., H. Fujimura, M. Matsumbura, T. Ueshima, T. Takahashi, and S. Senda, Analgesic action of dialkylaminoacylamino derivatives, I. (translated from Japanese), *J. Pharm. Soc. Japan*, *73*, 437–42 (1953).
358. Ott, A., Zur Kenntnis der neuen Arzneimittel: Phenacetin und Sulfonal, *Prager med. Wochschr.*, *13*, 432–34 (1888).
359. Ott, I., The antipyretics—acetphenetidin and antithermin, *J. Nervous Mental Disease*, *13*, 597–607 (1888).
360. Ott, I., *The modern antipyretics; their action, in health and disease*, 2nd ed., E. D. Vogel, Bookseller, Easton, Pa., 1892, 125 pp.
361. Ottoson, B.-G., Myanesin och compodyn vid efterbehandling av tonsillektomier, *Nord. med.*, *51*, 647 (1954).
362. Overlach, Zur Kenntnis einiger neuer Arzneimittel, *Centr. inn. Med.*, *45*, 1121–26 (1900).
363. Pagano, P. J., Migraine and the industrial physician. A review of the syndrome and report of the successful management of the problem in an industrial facility, *Ind. Med. Surg.*, *25*, 592–95 (1956).
364. Pagano, P. J., The migraine syndrome, *Med. Times*, *84*, 802–11 (1956).
365. Page, C. E., Measles and phenacetin: Which killed the patient—the disease or the treatment? *Med. News*, *65*, 577–78 (1894).
366. Paredes, J. M., and G. Lopez, Acción de los analgésicos antitérmicos sobre el corazón, *Farmacoterap. actual* (*Madrid*), *2*, 802–12 (1945).
367. Paterson, D. R., The untoward effects of antipyrin, acetanilide, and phenacetin, *Practitioner*, *51*, 241–49 (1893).
368. Pel, *Münch. med. Wochschr.*, *36*, 655 (1889).
369. Péréra, De la phénacétine, *Gaz. méd. d'Orient*, p. 43 (1888).
370. Pesce, Abst. from Turiner Kgl. Akad., *Deut. med. Wochschr.*, *14*, 1018 (1888).
371. Pesce, L., Osservazioni cliniche sulla Fenacetina, *Giorn. accad. med. Torino*, *36*, 122–25 (1888).

372. Pesce, L., and A. Assauto, Sulla paracetofenetidina, osservazioni cliniche *Riv. clin. (Milano)*, *28*, 201–28 (1889).

373. Piccinini, G. M., Variazioni visconsimetriche e crioscopiche del sangue per l'uso di antipirina fenacetina ed antifebbrina, *Arch. farmacol. sper.*, *12*, 193–209 (1911).

374. Piccinini, G. M., Gas du sang durant l'emploi de l'antipyrine, de la phénacétine et de l'antifébrine, *Arch. ital. biol.*, *58*, 449–54 (1912).

375. Piccinini, G. M., I gas del sangue durante l'uso di antipyrina, fenacetina e antifebbrina, *Arch. intern. pharmacodynamie*, *22*, 27–47 (1912).

376. Piccinini, G. M., Le variazioni dell'ossigeno mobile del sangue durante l'uso di Antipirina, Fenacetina e Antifebbrina, *Arch. farmacol. sper.*, *16*, 484–512 (1913).

377. Pierce, G. H., The general actions of phenacetine, *New Engl. Med. Monthly*, *9*, 440–44 (1889–90).

378. Pinder, J. L., and P. F. R. Venables, The British Pharmacopoeia test for readily carbonisable substances: I. Phenacetin, *Quart. J. Pharm. Pharmacol.*, *11*, 478–88 (1938).

379. Pitini, A., and S. Hamnett, Influenza degli antipiretici aromatici, *Arch. farmacol. terap.*, 11–24 (1899).

380. Pohle, K., and P. Dittrich, Vergleichende Untersuchungen über die analgetische Breite verschiedener Antipyretika bei Kombination mit Schlafmitteln. III. Mitteilung: Kombinationen mit Sulfonal, *Arch. exptl. Pathol. Pharmakol.*, *162*, 716–26 (1931).

381. Pohle, K., and W. Spieckermann, Vergleichende Untersuchungen über die analgetische Breite verschiedener Antipyretika bei Kombination mit Schlafmitteln. I. Mitteilung: Kombinationen mit Veronal, *Arch. exptl. Pathol. Pharmakol.*, *162*, 685–705 (1931).

382. Pohle, K., and F. Vogle, Vergleichende Untersuchungen über die analgetische Breite verschiedener Antipyretika bei Kombination mit Schalfmitteln. II. Mitteilung: Kombination mit Urethan, *Arch. exptl. Pathol. Pharmakol.*, *162*, 706–715 (1931).

383. Poljakov, V., On changes in blood in phenacetin poisoning (translated from Russian), *Medicinskoje Obozrjanil*, *72*, 721–33, (1909).

384. Popp, E., Das Phenacetin und seine Anwendung auf der würzburger medicinischen Klinik, Inaugural Dissertation (Univ. Würzburg), *Freiburg i. B.*, 1889, 54 pp.

385. Povorinskii, I. A., On phenacetin, *Zhur. Nervopatol. i Psikhiatrii*, *55*, 6–16 (1955).

386. Price, M. F., Phenacetine, *Southern Calif. Practitioner*, *4*, 329–33 (1889).

387. Rabenalt, H., Schmerzbekämpfung durch Commotional, *Med. Monatschr.*, *7*, 250–51 (1953).

388. Rabuske, J., Phenacetin gegen Migräne, *Deut. med. Wochschr.*, *14*, 767 (1888).

389. Rakieten, N., The effects of acetophenetidin, acetanilid, amidopyrine, aniline, and *para*-aminophenol on the rate of disappearance of ethyl alcohol from the blood, *Quart. J. Studies Alc.*, *3*, 97–102 (1942).

390. Reid, W. D., The heart in acetophenetidin (phenacetin) poisoning, *J. Am. Med. Assoc.*, *87*, 1036–37 (1926).

391. Reissmann, K., Schwere haemolytische "Randkörnchen." Anaemie durch chronische Phenacetinvergiftung infolge Antineuralgie-Tabletten-Süchtigkeit, *Med. Welt, 14,* 868–71 (1940).
392. Remsen, D., The use of *N*-acetyl-*p*-aminophenol, *Symposium on N-acetyl-p-aminophenol, The Institute for the Study of Analgesic and Sedative Drugs, Elkhart, Ind.,* 1952, pp. 59–61.
393. Renault, H., P. Rohrbach, and J. Dugniolle, Properiétés pharmacodynamiques du *N*-acétyl-*para*-aminophenol, métabolite de la phénacétine et de l'acétanilide, *Thérapie, 11,* 300–07 (1956).
394. Richelot, L.-G., P. Le Gendre, Luys, Grancher, H. Hallopeau, L.-H. Petit, and P. Chéron, La phénacétine, *L'Union médicale, 52,* 889–93 (1891).
395. Rifat, De la phénacétine, *Gaz. méd. d'Orient,* p. 42 (1888).
396. Rifat, De la phénacétine, *Gaz. méd. d'Orient,* p. 43 (1888).
397. Rifat, Traitement du rhumatisme aigu et blennorrhagique par la phénacétine à haute dose, *Bull. gén. thérap., 118,* 410–20 (1890).
398. Roback, G. S., L. R. Krasno, and A. C. Ivy, Effect of analeptic drugs on the somnifacient effect of seconal and antihistaminics as measured by the flicker fusion threshold, *J. Appl. Physiol., 4,* 566–74 (1952).
399. Robertson, F. D., The indiscriminate use of modern antipyretics, *Trans. Vermont Med. Soc.,* 205–12 (1894).
400. Roe, L., Phenacetine, *Brit. Med. J., 1888, I,* 1113.
401. Rohde, E., Aromatische Monamine, in Heffter, A., *Handbuch der experimentellen Pharmakologie,* Vol. I, Julius Springer, Berlin, 1923, pp. 1049–92.
402. Rohden, B., Phenacetin, *Deut. med. Wochschr., 14,* 366–67 (1888).
403. Rosen, R., Ueber Cosaprin und Phesin, zwei Ersatzmittel für Antifebrin und Phenacetin, *Therap. Monatsh., 13,* 156–58 (1899).
404. Rosenberger, P., Prophylaxe und Frühbehandlung von Grippe und Erkaltungskrankheiten in einem Industrieunternehmen während der letzten Jahre, *Deut. med. Wochschr., 79,* 1230–31 (1954).
405. Rovenstine, E. A., Clinical experiences with *N*-acetyl *p*-aminophenol, *Symposium on N-acetyl-p-aminophenol, The Institute for the Study of Analgesic and Sedative Drugs,* Elkhart, Ind., 1952, pp. 38–39.
406. Rumpf, Ueber das Phenacetin, *Berlin. klin. Wochschr., 25,* 457–61 (1888).
407. Russow, K. E., Ein Fall von tötlicher Phenacetinvergiftung, *St. Petersburger med. Wochschr., 33,* 33–35 (1908).
408. Ryan, R. E., Fiorinal for symptomatic treatment of nonvascular headache, *J. Missouri State Med. Assoc., 50,* 259–61 (1953).
409. Sajous, C. E. de M., The coal-tar derivatives *versus* opiates, *Monthly Cyclopedic Med. Bull., 3,* 156–59 (1910).
410. Sakanian, S. S., The effect of phenacetin on the reflex secretion of the stomach, *Farmakol. i Toxikol., 4,* 60 (1941).
411. Sandberg, F., The antipyretic and analgesic activity of some new *N*-substituted 5,5-diallylbarbiturates, *Svensk. Farm. Tidskr., 55,* 672–80 (1951).
412. Sandberg, F., The antipyretic and analgesic activity of some new *N*-substituted 5,5-diallylbarbiturates, *Svensk. Farm. Tidskr., 55,* 698–704 (1951).
413. Santarato, R., Azione dei farmaci sul metabolismo del piruvato nei feti

e negli animali giovani. III. Antipiretici e analgesici, *Boll. soc. ital. biol. sper.*, *29,* 630–32 (1953).

414. Sartorelli, E., and A. Quadrio, Anemia emolitica acuta da ingestione di fenacetina a scopo terapeutico, *Med. lavoro, 46,* 419–23 (1955).
415. Schaub, F., A. Bühlmann, and C. Maier, Blutschäden nach chronischem Phenacetinabusus, *Helv. Med. Acta, 20,* 428–32 (1953).
416. Schaub, F., A. Bühlmann, and C. Maier, Nebenerscheinungen und Folgen des chronischen Phenacetinabusus, *Schweiz. med. Wochschr.*, *83,* 626–29 (1953).
417. Schieffelin, W. H. and Co., *Clinical observations on the action of Phenacetine-Bayer,* New York, 1889, 8 pp.
418. Schieffelin, W. H. and Co., *Phenacetine-Bayer, antipyretic, analgesic, nerve sedative,* New York, 1891, 22 pp.
419. Schivardi, La fenacetina, *Gazz. ospediali, 9,* 473–74 (1888).
420. Schmahl, D. and A. Reiter, Fehlen einer cancerogenen Wirkung beim Phenacetin, *Arzneimittel-Forsch.*, *4,* 404–05 (1954).
421. Schmith K., and S. Madsen, Et tilfaelde af medicamentel forgiftning forarsaget af fenacetintabletter Ph. Dan. 48, *Ugeskrift Laeger, 112,* 1411–12 (1950).
422. Schødt, A., Et tilfaelde af Phenacetinforgiftning under Graviditel, *Ugeskrift Laeger, 100,* 859–61 (1938).
423. Schoffer, A., Über Phenacetin as Antineuralicum, Inaugural Dissertation, Strassburg, 1888, 34 pp.
424. Schub, C., Bietrag zur Kenntniss des Phenacetin als Nervinum, Inaugural Dissertation, Würzburg, *J. méd. Bordeaux,* 22 pp. (1888).
425. Schulze, E., Schmerzbekämpfung durch Gelonida-Suppositorien, *Med. Klin.* (*Munich*), *52,* 143 (1957).
426. Schweingruber, R., Probleme der chronischen Vergiftung mit kombinierten Phenacetinpräparaten, *Schweiz. med. Wochschr.*, *85,* 1162–66 (1955).
427. Schwensen, C. J., Anaemia haemolytica toxica. Phenacetinforgiftning, *Ugeskrift Laeger, 116,* 570–73 (1954).
428. Schwyzer, J., Die Fabrikation vom Guajakol und Phenazetin, *Pharm.* Z., *75,* 495–98; 509–10; 518–21 (1930).
429. Sears, T. P., Excessive use of empirin compound, *Rocky Mt. Med. J.*, *36,* 642 (1939).
430. Seidell, A., The solubility of acetanilide, phenacetine, caffeine and salol in several solvents, *J. Am. Chem. Soc.*, *29,* 1088–91 (1907).
431. Seller, D., Schmerzbekämpfung in der zahnärtzlichen Praxis, *Zahnärtzl.* Rundschau, *63,* 104 (1954).
432. Seitz, H., Über Erfahrungen mit D-Merzetten bei Miktionsstörungen, *Med. Monatschr.*, *11,* 31–32 (1957).
433. Selwyn, J. G., Heinz bodies in red cells after splenectomy and after phenacetin administration, *Brit. J. Haematol.*, *1,* 173–83 (1955).
434. Shlenker, M. A., Clinical observations of a new antipyretic, *Atlantic Med. Weekly*, *9,* 305–07 (1898).
435. Siegmund, E. A., R. A. Cadmus, and G. Lu, A method for evaluating both nonnarcotic and narcotic analgesics, *Proc. Soc. Exptl. Biol. Med.*, *95,* 729–31 (1957).

436. Siegmund, E. A., R. A. Cadmus, and G. Lu, Screening of analgesics, including aspirin-type compounds, based upon the antagonism of chemically induced "writhing" in mice, *J. Pharmacol, Exptl. Therap., 119,* 184 (1957).
437. Silver, D., I. W. Brown, Jr., and G. S. Eadie, Studies of experimental sulfhemoglobinemia, *J. Lab. Clin. Med., 48,* 79–91 (1956).
438. Sivadjian, J., Antipyrétiques et analgésiques, *Arch. intern. pharmacodynamie, 52,* 142–47 (1935–36).
439. Smith, D. L., M. C. D'Amour, and F. E. D'Amour, The analgesic properties of certain drugs and drug combinations, *J. Pharmacol. Exptl. Therap., 77,* 184–93 (1943).
440. Smith, J. N., and R. T. Williams, Studies in detoxication. 16. The metabolism of acetanilide in the rabbit, *Biochem. J., 42,* 538–44 (1948).
441. Smith, J. N., and R. T. Williams, Studies in detoxication. 22. The metabolism of phenacetin (*p*-ethoxyacetanilide) in the rabbit and a further observation on acetanilide metabolism, *Biochem, J., 44,* 239–42 (1949).
442. Smith, J. N., and R. T. Williams, Studies in detoxication. 23. The fate of aniline in the rabbit, *Biochem. J., 44,* 242–50 (1949).
443. Smith, J. N., and R. T. Williams, Studies in detoxication. 24. The metabolism of *p*-phenetidine (*p-ethoxyaniline*) with some observations on the anisidines (methoxyaniline), *Biochem. J., 44,* 250–55 (1949).
444. Smith, L. H., Jr., personal communication, 1956.
445. Smith, P. K., The changes in blood pigments of animals receiving large doses of acetanilid, sulfanilimide, and related compounds, *J. Pharmacol. Exptl. Therap., 66,* 33–34 (1939).
446. Smith, P. K., Changes in blood pigments associated with the prolonged administration of large doses of acetanilid and related compounds, *J. Pharmacol. Exptl. Therap., 70,* 171–78 (1940).
447. Smith, P. K., Progress report on "A search for inhibitors of poliomyelitis virus multiplication in tissue culture." National Foundation for Infantile Paralysis Grant CVRE97 (Jan. 1, 1953–June 30, 1953).
448. Smith, P. K., Progress report on "A search for inhibitors of poliomyelitis virus multiplication in tissue culture." National Foundation for Infantile Paralysis Grant CVRE97 (July 1, 1953–Dec. 31, 1953.)
449. Smith, P. K., Nonnarcotic analgesics and antipyretics. II. Drugs other than salicylates, in Drill, V. A., *Pharmacology in medicine; a collaborative textbook,* 2nd ed., McGraw-Hill Book Co., Inc. New York, Toronto, London, 1958, Chap. 21, 13 pp.
450. Smith P. K., C. Davison, and M. A. Sodd, Studies in the metabolism of *N*-acetyl-*p-aminophenol, Proc. Intern. Physiol. Congr., 20th Congr. Brussels,* 836–837 (1956).
451. Smith, P. K., and W. E. Hambourger, The ratio of the toxicity of acetanilid to its antipyretic activity in rats, *J. Pharmacol. Exptl. Therap., 54,* 346–51 (1935).
452. Snapper, I., Over Sulfhaemoglobinaemie, *Ned. Tijdschr. Geneesk., 66,* 2520–26 (1922).
453. Snapper, I., Phenacetin als Ursache für Sulfhämoglobinämie, *Deut. med. Wochschr., 51,* 648–50 (1925).

454. Soehring, K., and I. Tautz, Gesundheitsschäder durch akute und chronische Überdosierung von Acetylsalicylsäure und Phenacetin, *Med. Klin. (Munich)*, *51*, 1154–56 (1956).
455. Sokolov, D. A., On the influence of fever reducing agents (antipyrine, antifebrin, phenacetin, quinine and sodium salicylate) on the evaporation through the skin in normal and feverish children (translated from Russian), *Vrachebnoe Delo*, *14*, 385–86; 451–54; 606–11 (1893).
456. Sollmann, T., Comparative toxicity of local anesthetics and of antipyretics for earthworms, *J. Pharmacol. Exptl. Therap.*, *14*, 319–22 (1920).
457. Sollmann, T., *A manual of pharmacology and its application to therapeutics* and toxicology, 8th ed., W. B. Saunders Co., Philadelphia and London, 1957, xi, 1535 pp.
458. Sommer, A., Phenacetin bei der Behandlung des Typhus abdominalis, *Therap. Monatsh.*, *4*, 185–86 (1890).
459. Sonnenschein, R. R., and A. C. Ivy, Failure of oral antipyretic drugs to alter normal human pain thresholds, *J. Pharmacol. Exptl. Therap.*, *97*, 308–13 (1949).
460. Spalton, L. M., Production of codeine, *Lancet*, *270*, 339 (1956).
461. Specker, C. G. A., Contribution à l'étude de la phénacétine (variété *para*). Thèse de Doctorat en Médicine: Faculté de Médicine de Nancy, 1889, 70 pp.
462. Spühler, O., and H. U. Zollinger, Die chronisch-interstitielle Nephritis, *Z. klin. Med.*, *151*, 1–50 (1953).
463. Squier, T. L., and F. W. Madison, Primary granulocytopenia due to hypersensitivity to amidopyrine, *J. Allergy*, *6*, 9–16 (1934).
464. Squier, T. L., and F. W. Madison, Drug hypersensitivity as a cause of acute primary granulocytopenia, *Wisconsin Med. J.*, *34*, 175–78 (1935).
465. Stadie, W. C., Studies on blood changes in pneumococcus infections. An experimental study of the formation and fate of methemoglobin in the blood, *J. Exptl. Med.*, *33*, 627–40 (1921).
466. Stegagno, G., Antagonismo fra barbiturici cicloesenilici e acetilfenetidina. II. *Atti. soc. med. chir. Padova*, *18*, 313–16 (1940).
467. Stender, O., Verstärkung der lokalanästhesierenden Wirkung des Kokains und einiger seiner Ersatzmittel durch Paarung mit antipyretischen Giften, *Arch. exptl. Pathol. Pharmakol.*, *141*, 373–78 (1929).
468. Stern, R., Ueber das Verhalten der Wärmeregulation im Fieber und unter der Einwirkung von Antipyretica, *Z. klin. Med.*, *20*, 63–97 (1892).
469. Storozhevoj, M. G., On cases of phenacetin poisoning (translated from Russian), *Med. Obozvenije (Moscow)*, *71*, 791–98 (1908).
470. Strohschnieder, F., Vergleichende Untersuchungen über die schmerzstillende Wirkung einiger Antipyretica, Inaugural Dissertation, Münster, 1935, 35 pp.
471. Stroyberg, J., Et tilfaelde af forgiftning efter langvarig burg of tabl. codyli leo, *Ugeskrift Laeger*, *103*, 513 (1941).
472. Studer, A., and G. Zbinden, Experimenteller Beitrag zur Frage von Nierenschäden bei Abusus von phenazetinhaltigen Schmerzmitteln, *Experientia*, *11*, 450 (1955).

473. Suckling, C. W., Phenacetin, *Brit. Med. J., 1888, I,* 901.
474. Svirbely, J. L., Vitamin C studies in the rat. The effect of copper and various organic substances, *J. Biol. Chem., 131,* 233–41 (1939).
475. Swaminathan, S., A new method of synthesizing phenacetin and applied compounds, *Science and Culture, 12,* 199 (1946).
476. Tainter, M. L., E. G. Tainter, W. S. Lawrence, E. N. Neuru, R. W. Lackey, F. P. Luduena, H. B. Kirtland, Jr., and R. I. Gonzalez, Influence of various drugs on the threshold for electrical convulsions, *J. Pharmacol. Exptl. Therap., 79,* 42–54 (1943).
477. Thölen, H., Interstitielle Nephritis, *Schweiz. med. Wochschr., 84,* 963–67 (1954).
478. Thölen, H., J. Voegtli, H. Renschler, and A. Schaeffer, Ein Beitrag zur Genese der interstitiellen Nephritis, *Schweiz. med. Wochschr., 86,* 946–50 (1956).
479. Thomson, G. S., The antipyretic treatment of fevers, *Indian Med. Record, 8,* 253–54 (1895).
480. Tingley, W. K., Peculiar vaso-motor disturbance after the administration of phenacetine, *Med. Record, 42,* 341 (1892).
481. Tobey, G. L., Fatal poisoning by phenacetin in headache tablets, *Monthly Bull. State Board Health, Mass.,* p. 16 (Jan. 1908).
482. Torboli, A., Variazione dell'azione farmacologica della fenacetina in conseguenza dell'introduzione di un nucleo benzenico nella sua molecola, *Arch. sci. biol. (Italy), 22,* 71–73 (1936).
483. Traversa, G., Azione della fenacetina sui vasi sanguigni e sul disperdimento di calorico dalla pelle, *Progr. med., 5,* 161–69 (1891).
484. Trebing, J., Die Veranazetin-Äther-Narkose, *Therap. Monatsh., 30,* 242–44 (1916).
485. Trepte, G., Erfahrungen mit Neurasalonika, *Med. Klin. (Munich), 25,* 720 (1929).
486. Treupel, G. Beitrage zur Kenntniss der Antipyretica und Antalgica, *Deut. med. Wochschr., 21,* 222–24 (1895).
487. Treupel, G., Ueber die Kombination von Arzneimitteln, *Deut. med. Wochschr., 35,* 2014–15 (1909).
488. Tripold, F., Ueber die therapeutische Wirkung des Phenacetin und Thallin, *Wien. klin. Wochschr., 2,* 149–51 (1889).
489. Turner, F. C., personal communication.
490. Twombly, E. L., Epidemic influenza among the poor, *Boston Med. Surg. J., 122,* 270–72 (1890).
491. Ubaldi, A., Sull'aumento dell'acido solforico accoppiato nelle urine in seguito alla somministrazione di fenacetina. Azione tossica della fenacetina, *Riforma med., 6,* 752–53; 758–59 (1890).
492. Ubaldi, A., Sull'aumento dell'acido solforico accoppiato nelle urine in seguito a somministrazione di fenacetina. Azione tossica della fenacetina, *Bull. sci. med. Bologna, 1,* 498–502 (1890).
493. *United States Pharmacopeia,* 15th rev., Mack Publ. Co., Easton, Pa., 1955, lv, 1067 pp.

494. Valentin, Ein Fall von Phenacetinexanthem, *Therap. Monatsh., 2,* 330–31 (1888).
495. Van Loon, E. J., and B. B. Clark, Observations on the hematologic actions of acetanilid and acetophenetidin in the dog, *J. Lab. Clin. Med., 29,* 942–56 (1944).
496. Vegter, J. J. M., De invloed van eenige stabilisatoren op de ontleding van waterstofperoxyde en op het enzym katalase, *Pharm. Weekblad, 81,* 363–73 (1946).
497. Völker, R., Beitrag zur Behandlung des grippalen Infektes, *Medizinische, 1955,* 86–87.
498. Vollrath, W., Versuche am Menschen, die schmerzstillende Wirkung von Arzneimitteln und Kombinations-präparaten festzustellen, Inaugural Dissertation, Halle, 1934, 23 pp.
499. Von Oettingen, W. F., The aromatic amino and nitro compounds: Their toxicity and potential dangers, A review of the literature, *Natl. Insts. Health Bull.,* No. 271, (1941).
500. Von Oettingen, W. F., Phenol and its derivatives: the relation between their chemical constitution and their effect on the organism, *Natl. Insts. Health Bull.,* No. 190, (1949).
501. Waegner, A., Erfahrungen mit Complamin, einem neuen Kombinationspräparat, *Münch. med. Wochschr., 75,* 2050–51 (1928).
502. Waggoner, R. W., The choice of analgesics, *J. Am. Med. Assoc., 107,* 1049–52 (1936).
503. Wallenstein, S. L., and R. W. Houde, Clinical comparison of analgetic effectiveness of *N*-acetyl-*p*-aminophenol, salicylamide and aspirin, *Federation Proc., 13,* 414 (1954).
504. Warfvinge, F. W., Om acetfenetidin och acetanilid, *Hygiea, 50,* 554–66 (1888).
505. Warner, F., Phenacetine for the relief of pain, *Columbus Med. J., 24,* 374–77 (1900).
506. Warren, M. R., and H. W. Werner, The evaluation of antipyretics against pyrogen-induced fever, *J. Am. Pharm. Assoc., Sci. Ed., 35,* 256–59 (1946).
507. Washburn, W. H., and E. O. Kruger, Infra-red determination of aspirin, phenacetin, and caffeine, *J. Am. Pharm. Assoc., Sci. Ed., 38,* 623–25 (1949).
508. Weisman, S. J., Tension headache—treatment with an analgesic compound, *Am. Practitioner and Dig. Treatment, 6,* 1019–21 (1955).
509. Welsford, A. G., An overdose of phenacetin, *Brit. Med. J., 1911, I,* 1313.
510. Wenzel, D. G., J. L. Beal, and A. R. Haskell, The effect of antipyretics on the erythrocytic sedimentation rate of rats, *J. Am. Pharm. Assoc., Sci. Ed., 42,* 600–01 (1953).
511. Wesemann, W., Versuche am Menschen zur Auffindung wirksamer Kombinationen von Phenacetin und Dial, Thesis, Halle, 1931, 36 pp.
512. West, F. E., Note on the therapeutics of certain modern antipyretics, *Brooklyn Med. J., 7,* 325–65 (1893).
513. West, R. M., Two cases of phenacetin rash, *Lancet, 1895, I,* 91.
514. Westhaus, H., Akute Phenazetinvergiftung im Säuglingslater, *Kinderäztl. Prax., 21,* 9–11 (1953).

515. White, A. T., A case of acute cardiac dilatation, probably due to chronic phenacetin poisoning, *J. Trop. Med.*, *6*, 176–78 (1903).

516. Williams, F. H., Phenacetin, *Am. J. Med. Sci.*, 507–08 (1888).

517. Winogradow, A. P., Die Wirkung einiger Medikamente auf die Gallensekretion. Experimentelle Untersuchung. Phenacetin, *Z. Ges. exptl. Med.*, *43*, 584–604 (1924).

518. Winter, J. E., C. H. Richey, and H. G. Barbour, Magnesium oxide as an aid to the antipyretic action of phenacetin in dogs, *J. Pharmacol. Exptl. Therap.*, *38*, 343–47 (1930).

519. Wirz, G., Phenacetin als Nervinum, Inaugural Dissertation, Bonn, 1889, 29 pp.

520. Wittich, F. W., A recent preparation for the relief of vascular headache; preliminary report, *Quart. Rev. Allergy*, *10*, 90–3 (1956).

521. Wolf, D., Ueber klinische Erfahrungen mit Treupel-Suppositorien für Säuglinge, *Med. Klin. (Munich)*, *50*, 748 (1955).

522. Wolff, H. G., J. D. Hardy, and H. Goodell, Measurement of the effect on the pain threshold of acetylsalicylic acid, acetanilid, acetophenetidin, aminopyrine, ethyl alcohol, trichlorethylene, a barbiturate, quinine, ergotamine tartrate and caffeine; an analysis of their relation to the pain experience, *J. Clin. Invest.*, *20*, 63–80 (1941).

523. Wood, H. C., Jr., C. H. LaWall, H. W. Youngken, A. Osol, I. Griffith, and L. Gershenfeld, *The Dispensatory of the United States of America*, 22nd ed., plus supplement, J. B. Lippincott Co., Philadelphia and London, 1940, xix + 1894 + 76 pp.

524. Wood, H. C., Jr., and H. B. Wood, A study of the physiological action of phenacetin, *Univ. Med. Magazine, Philadelphia*, *13*, 360–62 (1900–01).

525. Wuhrmann, F., and B. Jasinski, Toxisch-hämolytische Anämie nach Phenacetin und Phenacetintoxikose, *Deut. med. Wochschr.*, *80*, 1632–34 (1955).

526. Yustoff, I. I., *Pathological-anatomical changes of blood and various organs in acute poisoning by phenacetin*, St. Petersburg, 1896, 86 pp.

527. Zadok, De la phénacétine, *Gaz. méd. d'Orient*, p. 44 (1888).

528. Zannas, De la phénacétine, *Gaz. méd. d'Orient, p.* 43 (1888).

529. Zollinger, H. U., Chronische interstitielle Nephritis bei Abusus von phenacetinhaltigen Analgetica (Saridon u.s.w.), *Schweiz. med. Wochschr.*, *85*, 746 (1955).

Index

Abdominal cramps, 128
Absorption, 8, 41, 114, 141, 142
Acetanilid, 1, 65
  analgesic action, 38–40, 42, 47, 48, 54, 56
  antipyretic action, 21, 23–28, 31, 33, 35
  cyanosis from, 3, 88–90, 93
  effect, on adrenals, 118
    on blood, 76–78, 82, 86, 99, 102, 107, 109, 110
    on central nervous system, 67, 68
    on enzymes, 120
    on hearing, 68
    on heart, 75
    on respiration, 111, 119
  habituation, 140
  metabolism, 141
  physical properties, 6, 17
  tolerance to, 138
  toxic effects, 121, 125, 130, 132, 133, 136, 139
N-Acetyl-*p*-aminophenol, analgesic action, 45, 46, 49, 51, 56–58, 143
  antipyretic action, 27, 29, 32, 36, 142
  effect, on blood, 77, 98, 99, 145, 146
    on cardiovascular system, 75, 144
    on central nervous system, 69, 70, 144
    on respiration, 112, 146
    on viruses, 63
  fate, 8–12, 14
  history, 3, 141
  metabolism, 16–19, 105, 109, 110, 142
  physical properties, 4, 5
  toxicity, 127, 134–136
N-Acetyl-*p*-phenetidine, 4
Acetylsalicylic acid (*see* Aspirin)
Acidosis, 114
Acylase, 17, 120
Addiction, 139, 140, 147
Adrenals, 117, 118
  effect on antipyretic action, 32
Adulteration, 6
Agranulocytosis (*see* Granulocytopenia)
Albuminuria, 124
Alcohol, 41, 42, 60, 118, 119
Allantoin, 114
Allergic reactions, 122, 130
Aluminum hydroxide, 44
p-Aminophenol, 13, 16, 17, 27, 89, 96
p-Aminopropiophenone, 105
Aminopyrine, analgesic action, 46, 48, 49, 53, 55
  antipyretic action, 31, 33, 34
  effect, on adrenals, 118
    on blood, 79, 80, 107, 108
    on hearing, 68
  synergism with cocaine, 61
  toxic effects of, 124, 126
Amobarbital (*see* also Barbiturates), 44, 55–57
Amphetamine, 44, 55, 56
Analgesic action, 24, 27, 28, 34, 37–59, 88, 101, 110, 112, 113, 138, 140, 143
Analytical methods, 7
Anemia, 79–81, 83, 115, 121, 131, 132, 139, 145, 146
  hemolytic, 78, 81–83, 89, 104, 126, 127
Anesthesia, local, 61
Aniline, 16, 71, 115
Antagonism to other drugs, 34, 67, 133, 134
Antihistamines (*see also individual antihistamines*), 43
Antikamnia, 71
Antipyretic action, 2, 20–39, 62, 120, 138, 142, 143

Antipyrine, 3, 5, 59, 77–79, 89–91, 95, 103, 109
  analgesic action, 37, 40, 54
  antipyretic action, 21, 23–28, 35, 36
  effect, on granulocytes, 110
    on hearing, 68
    on neuromuscular coordination, 68
    on skin, 121, 123
  local anesthetic effect, 61, 62
  toxic effects, 125, 126
Antiseptic action, 62
Anxiety, 60
Appetite, 2, 29, 64, 117, 122, 137, 139, 142
Arthritis, 29, 39, 42, 43, 45, 53, 57, 59, 88, 102, 143
Ascorbic acid, 44, 61
  in organs, 116–118
  in treatment of toxicity, 79, 132
Aspirin, 8, 29, 41–44, 56, 61, 67, 71, 72, 80,81, 91, 102, 103, 107, 110, 124, 126, 130, 131, 134, 139, 143
  analgesic action, 45–48, 52, 53, 57
  antipyretic action, 30, 31, 33–35
  effect, on hearing, 68
    on neuromuscular coordination, 68
    on vibratory threshold, 69
    on vision, 68
  habit formation, 140
  synergism with, 55
  toxic effects, 132, 133
Ataxia, 69
Atherosclerosis, 72
Atropine, 139

Bactericidal action, 62
Barbital (*see also* Barbiturates), 40–42, 46, 54, 60, 62, 124
  antagonism by, 32, 48, 133
  synergism with, 33
Barbiturates (*see also specific barbiturates*), 43, 80, 107, 124, 130, 142, 143
  antagonism of, 133
  synergism with, 36
Basic metabolic rate, effect on, 119
Belladonna, 44
Benzyl benzoate, 43
Bile, 116
Bioflavonoids, 56
Bismuth, 86, 90
Blood, cell volume, 83
  cells (*see* Erythrocytes; Granulocytopenia; Leucocytes; Reticulocytes)
  dyscrasia, 81, 92
  glucose, 118
  pigments (*see* Methemoglobin; Sulfhemoglobin)
  pressure, 70–76, 112, 115, 134, 144
  vessels, 35, 72, 74, 75
Bone marrow, 78–80, 109, 130, 144, 146
Brain, 11, 14, 142
Bromides, 107, 130
Bronchitis, 23, 29, 129

Caffeine, 8, 29, 34, 35, 42–44, 48, 54, 55, 57, 60, 61, 64, 69, 71, 77–81, 86, 87, 89–91, 93, 95, 103, 107, 109, 110, 114, 124, 129, 131, 143
  in treatment of toxicity, 125, 132
Calcium lactate, 55
Camphor, 87
Carbhemoglobin, 105
Carbohydrate metabolism, 116
Carbon dioxide, 118, 119
Carbonic anhydrase, 114
Carbromal, 32, 48
Carcinogenicity, 116
Catalase, 119
Central nervous system, 3, 22, 37, 67–70, 134, 142
Cerebrospinal fluid, 9, 14, 142
Chills, 22, 23, 26, 28
p-Chloroacetanilid, 6, 94, 96
Cholesterol, 117
Choline esterase, 120
Circulation, 29, 142

Citrate, 8, 41, 142
Cocaine, 61
Codeine, 8, 29, 41, 42, 55–57, 60, 61, 80, 90, 94, 124, 126, 131, 139, 143
  analgesic action, 45
  antagonism of, 134
  synergism with, 54
Colds, 43, 129, 140
Collapse, 2, 70, 84, 88, 93, 126, 142,
Color index, 83
Conjugation, 18
  glucuronic acid, 15–18
  sulfate, 15–17, 119
Constipation, 139
Convulsions, 64, 65, 67, 70, 87, 135, 139
Coordination, 68
Cyanosis, 2, 3, 29, 75, 79, 80, 96, 100–102, 105, 115, 125–129, 132, 139, 140, 142, 145, 146
Cystitis, 29

Deacetylation, 18
Death, 128, 129, 147
De-ethylation, 17, 18
Dependence, physical, 140
Desoxyephedrine, 62, 67
Diallylbarbituric acid, 32, 48, 54, 57, 67, 107
Diarrhea, 86, 88, 104, 113, 128
Dibenzyl aminoethanol, 44
Diethylamino-ethyldiphenylpropyl-acetate, 17
3,3-Diethyl-2,4-dioxotetrahydro-pyridine, 114
Digitalis, 70, 72, 75, 128, 131, 139
Dihydromorphinone, 40
Dilaudid, 42, 43
Dimethylaminophenazone, 29, 42, 43, 124
Dinitrophenol, 107
Diphenhydramine, 60
Distribution in tissues, 11
Dovers powder, 128
Dysentery, 24, 128, 129
Dysmenorrhea, 42, 43, 70, 72
Dyspnea, 72

Edema, 71, 122, 124, 128
Effervescent base, 10, 11
Electro-cutaneous sensitivity, 68
Enteric fever, 27
Enzyme systems (*see also specific enzymes*), 119, 120, 127, 144, 146
Ergotamine tartrate, 44
Erysipelas, 23, 92
Erythema, 123
Erythrocytes, 11, 76–83, 105
Ether, 61, 73
p-Ethoxyacetanilid, 4
Eucaine, 61
Excretion, 7, 13, 14, 115, 119

Fevers, 1–3, 59, 85, 110, 118, 121, 129, 138, 142
Formulas, structural, 4

Gastrointestinal tract, 8, 14, 131, 141
Glucose, 17, 118, 132
Glucose-6-phosphate dehydrogenase, 82
Glucuronide, 15–18, 141
Glycosuria, 114
Granulocytopenia, 106–110, 130

Habituation, 139, 140, 147
Hay-fever, 61
Headache, 24, 29, 37–40, 42–45, 53, 58, 64, 65, 70, 76, 78, 79, 86, 90, 91, 95, 102, 113, 121, 124, 125, 128, 129, 138–140, 143
Hearing, 64, 68, 70, 144
Heart, 2, 27, 28, 70–73, 75, 76, 89, 111, 118, 129, 131, 144
  rate, 65, 70, 72–75, 126, 131
Heinz bodies, 80, 81
Hematin, 76
Hematuria, 112
Hemoglobin, 76–80, 82–84, 92, 100, 101, 104

Hemolysis, 76, 81, 82, 128
Hemorrhage, 123, 131
Herpes zoster, 39, 43
Hexabarbital, 62
Hydrogen sulfide, 100
p-Hydroxyacetanilid, 4
Hydroxylamine, 17
Hyoscyamus, 107
Hypnotic effect, 22, 34, 49, 54, 60, 62, 70, 143

Idiosyncrasy, 122–124, 130
Infection, 142
Influenza, 27, 28, 39–43, 45, 61, 108, 111, 129, 143
Insomnia, 24, 44, 60
Intestine, 73, 104, 118, 120
Ipecac, 128
Iron, 79, 80, 82, 100, 127, 132, 144
Isobutylallylbarbituric acid, 44
Isonipecaine, 80
Isopropylantipyrine, 78, 79, 94, 95, 104, 113, 114
Isopropylphenazone, 29, 43
Itching, 121, 122

Jaundice, 115

Kidney, 38, 73, 113–115, 131
  function, 112, 114, 115, 119, 146

Lactophenine, 62
Lactylphenetidin, 44
LD_{50}, 92, 133, 135
Lead poisoning, 128
Lethal dose, 74, 92, 133, 135
Leucocytes, 76, 106–110, 113, 128, 130, 145, 146
Leukemia, 64
Liver, 113, 115, 118–120, 128, 131, 146
  function, 100, 101, 116, 146
  glycogen, 116, 118
Liver extract, 79
Lung, 89, 129

Magnesium, 17, 34, 42, 44
Malaria, 27, 37, 40, 128
Measles, 128
Mental functions, 2, 3, 22, 40, 64, 65, 67, 70, 79, 110, 126, 139, 144
Metabolism, 15–19
Methemoglobin, 16, 75, 80, 90, 91–105, 108, 113, 131, 132, 145, 147
Methoxyaceto-*p*-phenetidin, 27,
N-Methyl-cyclohexenyl-methyl-barbiturate, 133
Migraine, 22, 29, 37–39, 41, 42, 44, 45, 70, 78, 85, 123, 143
Morphine, 37, 42, 46, 60, 87, 90, 94, 113, 126, 128, 129, 139
Muscle, 117
  glycogen, 116, 118

Nausea, 2, 3, 22, 29, 61, 65, 70, 104, 142, 144
Neoarsphenamine, 108
Neocinchophen, 30, 31
Nephritis (*see also* Kidney), 2, 29, 112–114
Neuralgia, 37–40, 42, 43, 86, 87, 122, 123, 143
Nicotinamide, 17
Nicotine, 42
Nux vomica, 70

Opium, 40, 128
Otitis, 29, 106
Overdosage, 129, 130
Oxygen, capacity, 105
  consumption, 117, 118
  content, 83
  tension, 103

Pain, 86–88, 122, 129
  threshold, 46, 47, 50, 53
Pancreatic enzymes, 8
Papaverine, 42, 43
Penicillin, 44, 61
Peralga, 107
Peritonitis, 40

Persedon, 113, 114
Perspiration, 2, 20, 21, 23–25, 28, 37, 38, 65, 119, 122, 129, 139
Phenacetin, 4, 88
Phenemal, 44
Phenetidin, 9, 11, 12, 15–19, 97, 142
Phenetsal, 41
Phenobarbital, 8, 29, 40, 43, 61, 90, 91, 95
1-Phenyl-2,3-dimethyl-4-isopropyl-5-pyrazolone, 114
1-Phenyl-2,3-dimethyl-4-methyl-aminopyrazalone-*N*-methane sulfonate, 56
Phenyldimethylpyrazine, 29, 42
Phenyldimethylpyrazolone, 29, 44
Phenylquinoline carboxylic acid, 43
Phenylquinolinic acid, 41
Phenyl salicylate, 28, 40, 68
Phenyltoloxamine diacetate, 61
  dihydrogen citrate, 43
Phosphatase, 120
Phosphorylation, 120, 146
Physical-chemical properties, 4–6
Plasma concentration, 8, 9, 11, 14, 142
Pleurisy, 21, 40
Pneumonia, 2, 21, 23, 24, 27–29, 40, 61, 129, 131, 136
Poliomyelitis, 63, 144
Potassium sulfide, 105
Pregnancy, 90
Primaquine, 81, 82
Propadrine, 42, 72
Protein, binding, 11, 14, 142
  digestion, 119
  effect on, 114
Pruritus, 123
Psychiatric patients, 60
Puerperal fever, 23
Pulse rate, 22, 71, 72, 75, 125, 126
Pyruvate decarboxylase, 120

Quinine, 23, 28, 29, 40, 42, 44, 61, 68, 80, 110, 121, 128

Reacetylation, 18
Red blood cells (*see* Erythrocytes)
Respiration, 71, 75, 110–112, 125, 126, 135, 139, 146
Respiratory infections, 44, 61, 113
Reticulocytes, 78–80, 83
Rheumatism, 27, 28, 37–40, 45, 59, 129

Salicylamide, 43, 55, 56, 60, 61, 67, 133
Salicylates (*see also* Aspirin), 23, 26, 28, 48, 141
  analgesic action, 38, 40, 46, 143
  effect on enzymes, 120, 141, 146
Salivation, 67
Sciatica, 37–40, 43, 45, 143
Seasickness, 61
Sedative action, 54, 60, 62
Sedimentation rate, 82, 83
Serum viscosity, 118
Skin, 20, 35, 59, 108, 121–124, 128, 147
Smoking, 54
Sodium bicarbonate, 8, 125, 132
Speech, 130
Spleen, 115–118, 128, 146
Stomach, 8, 40, 73, 100, 118
Strychnine, 67
Sulfanilamide, 90
Sulfate, conjugation, 11, 15–18, 119
Sulfhemoglobin, 79, 91, 94, 95, 97, 99–105, 108, 126, 145
Sulfonal, 30, 46
Sulfur, 100–102, 105
Synergism, 33–35, 48, 61, 134

Tabes, 37, 39, 42, 101, 131
Temperature regulation, 26, 32, 34, 118
Thrombocytopenia purpura, 80
Tolerance, 138
Toxic effects, 130, 147
Toxicity, 6
Tremor, 130, 139
Trinitroluene, 105
Triphosphopyridine nucleotide, 17

Tuberculosis, 2, 20–24, 27, 37, 45, 62, 89, 92, 143
Tumor, 38, 40, 63, 129, 144
Typhoid fever, 2, 20–24, 27, 29, 39, 45, 59, 85, 121, 129
Typhus, 2, 23, 26, 40, 85, 122

Urethane, 33, 46, 73
Uterus, 120

Vasomotor system, 75
Verdiglobin, 103, 104
Vertigo, 3, 70, 144
Vision, 68
Vitamin B_{12}, 132
Vomiting, 2, 3, 29, 61, 65, 70, 71, 104, 113, 128, 129, 139, 142, 144

Weight, body, 117, 137
White blood cells (*see* Leucocytes)
Whooping cough, 59, 61
Withdrawal symptoms, 140, 147